250 Medical Questions Answered

About the author

Dr Ann Robinson is a GP, medical columnist for *The Guardian* and *Essentials*, and has done online consultations for Freeserve. She is author of *The Which? Guide to Women's Health*, which also received a commendation from the British Medical Association. She is married and has three children.

Acknowledgements

The author and publisher would like to thank Dr Harry Brown for his comments on the text. Thanks too to the research staff at Consumers' Association for their contributions.

250 Medical Questions Answered

Dr Ann Robinson

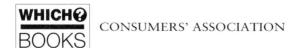

CONSUMERS' ASSOCIATION

Which? Books are commissioned by
Consumers' Association and published by
Which? Ltd, 2 Marylebone Road, London NW1 4DF
Email: books@which.net

Distributed by The Penguin Group:
Penguin Books Ltd, 80 Strand, London WC2R 0RL

First edition January 2002
Bound in new cover June 2004

Copyright © 2002 Which? Ltd

British Library Cataloguing in Publication Data
A catalogue record for *250 Medical Questions Answered* is available from the British Library

ISBN 0 85202 964 0

For a full list of Which? books, please call 0800 252100, access our website at www.which.net, or write to Which? Books, Freepost, PO Box 44, Hertford SG14 1SH

Editorial and production: Alethea Doran, Vicky Fisher, Robert Gray, Nithya Rae, Barbara Toft
Index: Marie Lorimer
Original cover concept by Sarah Harmer
Cover photograph by David Arky/getty images

Typeset by Saxon Graphics Ltd, Derby
Printed and bound in Great Britain by Creative Print and Design, Wales

Contents

★ An asterisk next to the name of an organisation in the text indicates that the address or web site can be found in this section

Introduction

We all worry about our health, possibly more than is good for us. With the burgeoning number of web sites, magazines, books and columns in newspapers on every health topic imaginable, we are all better informed and perhaps therefore more concerned about our health than we ever were. So why another book on health?

The answer is simple: some problems are too embarrassing to disclose to friends or a partner, too worrying to mention to a doctor, or just too toe-curlingly revolting to share with a soul. Even in the anonymity of cyberspace we may not be able to face up to certain issues or find medical advice that is reliable or relevant to us. *The Which? Guide to Personal Health* seeks to reassure readers; where necessary, it urges them to seek professional help.

The reasons we find it difficult to talk about certain subjects to a doctor are varied. One of the main ones is what he or she will think of us. People who suffer from smelly feet, body odour or bad breath, for example, may feel that they will be looked down on by their GP. Others may worry that they will be considered promiscuous if they have a sexually transmitted disease or want to terminate a pregnancy. Those with a dependence on alcohol, nicotine, drugs or food may feel they will be dismissed as time-wasters whose problems are self-inflicted. However, health professionals are trained not to be judgmental, and nasty smells, vaginal disorders and addictions are all in a day's work for most doctors and nurses.

Another reason we may not want to discuss a problem with our doctor is because we have had a bad experience in the past. Perhaps we were treated brusquely, or examined roughly, or felt that our privacy was not being respected. No one should ever be made to feel this way and if you are, discuss your feelings with your doctor. If you are not satisfied with the response, consider complaining formally or at least moving to another practice or specialist.

A third reason is that most of us are shy of talking about and showing our bottoms and genitals. We may find it easier to look for advice in a book than to drop our trousers or take off a bra in front of a doctor. But no written information can be a substitute for a face-to-face consultation.

Another factor that may stop us from visiting a doctor is that we may not know what our condition – or indeed the relevant part of the body – is called. However, this should not cause us to feel ill at ease. It is always clearer to describe symptoms in simple language when speaking to a health professional, and he or she should do the same. The use of plain English in place of ancient Latin and Greek would benefit everyone. This book includes glossaries explaining commonly used terms.

We may find some subjects to be so painful or frightening to talk about that we may prefer to look in a book than say the words out loud. Sexual abuse in childhood, bullying and rape need to be reported and dealt with, but it may be very hard to summon up the courage to do so. Finding a lump in the breast or testicle may frighten us so much that we may pretend it is not there. But as this book points out, not all lumps are cancerous, and not all cancers are death sentences by any means – most can be treated and many are curable, but only with prompt and appropriate attention.

Sometimes, we may not want to seek medical advice because we think that nothing can be done to help us. Some conditions, such as testicular pain, a blocked nose or blushing, are hard to treat success-fully but that does not mean that we should not look for a solution. At the very least, the doctor may be able to reassure us that there is no serious underlying cause; at best we may be given useful advice.

The Which? Guide to Personal Health tries to answer many of the sorts of questions that people write to medical columnists about, but are often reluctant to mention in their GP's surgery. Clearly, it cannot be comprehensive, but if you find that your particular con-cern is not dealt with, remember that the aim of the guide is to emphasise that no issue is too embarrassing to seek advice for. So if it makes you go and talk to your GP – to air and share your worry, rather than bury it – the book will have achieved its goal.

Chapter 1

Lifestyle and general health worries

Life expectancy in the UK is higher than ever before, and we all hope to live out our allotted years without pain or serious illness. However, very few of us are entirely free from worry about our health. Compared with previous generations, our experience of early death is limited, so the premature illnesses or deaths of our contemporaries frighten us inordinately, and we may harbour fears about our own fate. It is hard not to imagine that some nagging symptom could be a sign of something serious, or worry that we might be at risk of a fatal illness because it has afflicted other members of the family.

Modern life is often busy and stressful, which can have an effect on the way we treat ourselves. At the same time there is a pressure to be successful and attractive. Some of us feel very unhappy about some aspect of our lifestyle, body or appearance, which we would like to change but either lack the confidence to pursue or do not know how to.

All these concerns can be hard to talk about with a doctor. We might feel that the problem is not the sort of thing we can express easily, or that it is unlikely to elicit sympathy in a rushed ten-minute consultation, particularly if there are no obvious symptoms. A physical debility may be affecting or undermining our life but might not seem specific enough to be easily solved by the doctor. Or, we may be worried about someone we care about, and do not know how to help.

This chapter first gives guidance about changing the way you look, in terms of both weight loss and cosmetic surgery procedures. It offers suggestions about how to deal with drinking, smoking and drug-taking, and where to go for further help. Advice is given about possible causes of chronic tiredness or debility, help for insomnia, and the best way to go about preventing and detecting serious diseases such as cancer.

Obesity

Q *I am 52 years old and am seriously overweight: I weigh 21 stone [133kg]. I have just developed diabetes, and already have high blood pressure and asthma. I really need to lose ten stone and need help to do it. I have been down all the usual routes of diets and classes, but constantly fail. Is there anything that will help me to lose the weight?*

A You will need a lot of patience and encouragement if you are to achieve lasting weight loss. Rather than thinking in terms of losing ten stone (64 kg) – a daunting prospect for even the most committed dieter – you will probably be more motivated to think in terms of making small manageable changes to your diet and level of physical activity, and aim to lose, say, 2–3lbs (1–1.5kg) a week.

Anyone in your position should try the following practical steps.

- Keep a food diary for one week, not changing anything about the way or amount you eat, but being scrupulously honest. Admitting what you eat is the first step to being in control of your eating. People who show the commitment needed to keep an honest and complete food diary for a week tend to be able to change their eating patterns and lose weight over a long period. People who dismiss the idea as a waste of time seem to be the ones who are not really motivated.
- Having kept the diary for a week, analyse what you are eating and when. You really need to cut out around 500 calories a day to lose 1lb (0.5kg) of fat a week. Continual snacking, eating straight from the fridge or breadbin without sitting down to eat, late-night eating and finishing off children's food are all ways of piling on extra calories. Most of us can easily cut out 500 calories a day by eating planned meals, preferably in the company of other people, three times a day, with only fruit in between.
- Every day, you need to do some sort of physical exercise. It might be walking to the shops, walking to collect children from school, or joining an aqua-aerobics class at the local pool – it does not matter what it is so long as it lasts for at least 20 minutes and

makes you feel your heart has speeded up or that you are a bit out of breath as a result.

- Book an appointment with your GP and take someone with you if you feel it will help. You should be referred to a dietician, and you may want to try taking the drug orlistat (Xenical – see page 14), if your GP thinks it would be suitable for you. Referral to a specialist in hormones (an endocrinologist) may be considered if you find that your weight is not dropping despite dieting – although in practice it is very rare to find a hormonal cause of excess weight.

The British Heart Foundation★ can provide helpful information and advice.

Blood pressure

'Blood pressure' refers to the pressure of blood in the arteries. The higher your blood pressure, the greater your risk of developing damaged arteries, which can lead to heart problems and strokes (see box later in this chapter). High blood pressure occurs when blood flows through arteries that are narrowed because of various factors such as smoking and high cholesterol. High blood pressure can be lowered by making changes to your lifestyle, for example, by changing your diet, exercising or losing weight. If necessary, blood pressure can also be lowered with tablets.

Q *I am 16 years old and overweight. I weigh 15 stone [95kg] and have only been able to lose half a stone in the past three to four months. I have tried dieting many times and also tried missing out meals but it doesn't help. I don't have the money to join a diet group and am too nervous about going to see my doctor. I am also getting teased at school. What can I do to lose weight?*

A You have taken the first and most important step to getting on top of your problem by acknowledging it. Make an appointment with a doctor whom you already know and take a parent or a mature friend with you for moral support if you want. The doctor will probably ask you about your eating patterns, how much exercise you take, and perhaps whether there are any emotional problems that could be causing you to overeat. You could ask for some blood tests – to check what your cholesterol level is, whether your thyroid is underactive, and what your hormone levels are. These will help to find out whether you have an underlying problem contributing to your weight. For instance, if your thyroid is underactive, a daily tablet can help to make the weight fall off you.

Cholesterol

Cholesterol is one of the fats found in all human and animal tissues. It is carried around the body by the blood. Some cholesterol comes directly from food, and some is made by the liver.

High cholesterol levels cause fatty deposits to build up inside blood vessels. Eventually the vessels can become blocked and blood cannot flow through them. This is particularly likely to happen in the narrow vessels that supply blood to the muscle of the heart – the coronary arteries – which may cause damage to the heart and can cause angina or a heart attack.

High blood cholesterol is usually the result of eating too much fat. It can also be caused by not getting enough exercise. Occasionally, high cholesterol runs in the family, and in these circumstances it is because the body does not cope well with normal amounts of cholesterol in food. A blood test can identify high cholesterol levels. You can lower your cholesterol level by eating a low-fat diet, doing regular exercise – which increases the 'good' component of cholesterol, called high density lipoprotein (HDL) – or with certain drugs, the most common group of which are known as statins.

If you can show that you can lose some weight on a calorie-controlled diet, as you already have done, you may be prescribed orlistat (Xenical – see below), which can help you lose weight more easily than just dieting.

Ultimately, it is going to be a question of controlling what you eat and increasing the amount of exercise you do. Your GP will probably be able to refer you (with whoever cooks at home) to a dietician, and you may want to look in at your local sports centre to see if there are any reasonably priced exercise classes or times when you can go for a swim. Alternatively, an early morning jog or cycle ride around the block is free.

Thyroid disorders

The thyroid gland is the same shape and size, and sits in the same position, as a bow tie. It is controlled by a hormone called TSH (thyroid-stimulating hormone), produced by the brain, which 'instructs' the thyroid gland to produce thyroid hormones. These hormones (the main one is thyroxine) circulate in the bloodstream and are responsible for driving many of the body's functions. For reasons that are not well understood, women are more prone than men to having too much or too little thyroid hormone.

Having an underactive thyroid is like having your car engine tuned too low: your whole body operates below par. This may result in weight gain, lethargy, shortness of breath, puffy ankles, feeling cold the whole time, thin hair, and heavy periods in women. Diagnosis is confirmed by blood test. The treatment, which must continue for life, consists in taking a daily tablet to replace the thyroxine.

Having an overactive thyroid is like having your car engine tuned too high: your whole body is in overdrive. This may result in weight loss, shaking hands, sweating, palpitations, irritability and infrequent periods in women. In some cases the eyes may look bulging and staring. Diagnosis is confirmed by blood test and further tests may be necessary to determine the underlying cause. Treatment initially involves drugs to lower the thyroxine level and to control the symptoms. Then the options are: surgery to remove part of the thyroid gland, or a dose of radioactive iodine, which is absorbed by the thyroid gland and results in its partial destruction. Both treatments may be overeffective, resulting in too little thyroxine and requiring medication, as in the case of an underactive thyroid, to adjust the level.

Diabetes

Diabetes – or to give it its full name, diabetes mellitus – is a condition in which the amount of glucose (sugar) in the blood is too high. This is because the body's method of converting glucose into energy is not working as it should. Normally, a hormone called insulin helps the glucose to enter the cells, where it is used as fuel by the body. Insulin carefully regulates the amount of glucose in the blood, by controlling the rate at which it is taken up by the cells. It is made by a gland called the pancreas, which lies just behind the stomach.

We obtain glucose from food, either from sweet foods or from the digestion of starchy foods such as bread or potatoes. The liver can also make glucose. After a meal, the blood glucose level rises, which stimulates the pancreatic cells to release insulin into the blood. When the blood glucose level falls – for example, during physical activity – the rate of insulin production falls. Insulin, therefore, plays a vital role in stopping the blood glucose from rising too high or sinking too low. High glucose levels in the blood can be damaging to the blood vessels and to various organs such as the heart, kidneys and eyes.

There are two main types of diabetes:

- type-1 diabetes, also known as insulin-dependent diabetes
- type-2 diabetes, also known as non-insulin-dependent diabetes.

Type-1 diabetes develops when there is a severe lack of insulin in the

---

Q *I am very fat. I am always trying to diet but it doesn't seem to make any difference. Should I try the new fat-busting drug, Xenical?*

A It depends a bit on how fat you are and what else you have tried. You are considered to be obese if your body mass index (BMI, which is weight in kilograms divided by height in metres squared – see chart on page 16) is more than 30. If you have tried at least three months of a sensible diet, tried to exercise, and sought some help from a GP or dietician, all to no avail, then orlistat (Xenical) may indeed be a good idea. This drug stops you absorbing about a third of the fat you eat and makes it pass straight through your gut. Your body because most or all of the cells in the pancreas that produce it have been destroyed. This type of diabetes usually appears in people under the age of 30, often in childhood. It is treated by insulin injections and a controlled diet.

Type-2 diabetes develops when the body can still produce some insulin, although not enough for its needs, or when the insulin that the body produces does not work properly. This type of diabetes usually appears in people over the age of 30. It is treated by controlled diet alone – to ensure that the blood sugar levels do not rise too high – or by a combination of diet and drugs that stimulate the pancreatic cells. Symptoms of diabetes include an unusually high degree of thirst or need to urinate. Tiredness or lethargy is likely to be felt with untreated diabetes, although tiredness is a common problem that could well be the result of other causes. More unusual symptoms include blurring of the vision, recurrent infections (because diabetes lowers your immunity), and weight loss, especially among younger women. Some of the excess glucose is passed in the urine and so can be detected by a simple urine test. Blood tests that check blood glucose levels are a more accurate measure.

Type-1 diabetes may be associated with other auto-immune diseases (i.e. in which the body attacks itself), or be caused by genetic predisposition, or possibly triggered by external factors such as a viral infection. Type-2 diabetes has a stronger inherited tendency, and is often triggered by obesity.

GP is not supposed to prescribe it unless you can show commitment by losing 2.5kg over four weeks, without drugs.

On average, out of 100 very overweight people who try to stick to a low-calorie diet and take more exercise, 15 will lose 10 per cent of their total weight in a year. When dieting and exercise are combined with Xenical, this goes up to 30 out of the 100. So the drug is no guarantee of weight loss, but it can boost your efforts.

The flip-side of Xenical is that it may cause bloating, a very strong urge to defecate, and oily stools that will not flush away. And since not everyone who tries it loses weight, it can be disappointing. The drug is licensed for use for up to two years; however, it should be stopped after three months if you have not lost 5 per cent of your body weight by that time. It is not a long-term option, therefore – it can be a very useful kickstart to your weight loss, but the acid test is whether you manage to adjust your lifestyle so that any weight you lose stays off. New drugs that work on the brain to stop food craving

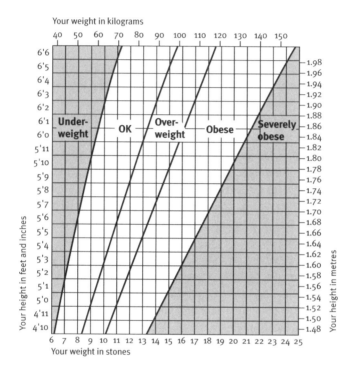

Body mass index (BMI)

and help to suppress appetite are being developed (see below). They are similar to antidepressants and therefore work very differently from Xenical.

Q *I'm obese and have heard of a new slimming tablet that can help suppress my appetite. When I tried Xenical I found that it had unpleasant side-effects. Is this new drug different?*

A There is a new appetite-suppressant pill called Reductil (sibu-tramine hydrochloride monohydrate) to add to the range of options for the extremely overweight and it does work in a different way to Xenical. It is available on prescription for those who are obese and for whom diet and exercise alone are not working. Reductil is one of a group of drugs developed initially as antidepressants, and works by increasing the brain's levels of circulating chemicals known as noradrenaline and serotonin. These chemicals are said to enhance signals in your brain telling you that you are full up, so you eat less than you would have. The side-effects are usually mild and temporary, and could take the form of a headache, insomnia, constipation or a dry mouth. The main risk with the drug is that it can substantially raise your blood pressure, thereby increasing your risk of heart attacks and strokes. For this reason, you should not take it if you already have high, uncontrolled blood pressure; if you do take it, make sure you have regular blood pressure checks and discontinue the drug if your pressure starts to climb. Whether Reductil is effective and what its effects are in the long term remain to be seen.

Cosmetic surgery

Q *I am finding it very hard to come to terms with the visible ageing of my body, and am seriously considering surgery to improve the appearance of my wrinkled, sagging face and neck. Can you tell me a bit about it and offer any advice?*

A As we age, our skin gets thinner and less elastic, the underlying facial muscles sag, and the fat that pads our cheeks while we are younger slips down around the jaw. We all age at different rates, depending on our genetic makeup and lifestyle – the effects of sun and smoking, in particular, accelerate the ageing effect. Whether we see the result as a face full of character – with experiences and a story to tell – or as a ravaged face that needs fixing, depends on us.

Hundreds of thousands of people in the UK have had some cosmetic surgery, in the belief that it will make them feel more confident and better about themselves. About 90 per cent are women, and about 90 per cent of the operations are to reverse signs of ageing. It may be worth fixing your wrinkles if they are really the one thing that is preventing you from being happy. However, some people have major surgery only to find that they then fixate on something else, because the real problem is low self-esteem caused by other factors – ones that could be better tackled by counselling than by surgery.

Bear in mind that no surgery, even if it is a minor procedure, is risk-free. Infections and complications (such as haemorrhaging and scarring) may occur, and the outcome may not be successful or quite what you wanted. Ask yourself the following questions before you decide to go ahead with cosmetic surgery.

- Once I have this operation, will I be happy with the way I look?
- Am I prepared for the fact that the operation can cause damage?
- Am I being realistic about the likely result? (Have I seen photos or computer-generated pictures of the likely outcome?)
- Am I satisfied that the surgeon is experienced in doing this particular operation, and is a member of a recognised professional body? (See below)
- Do I know how much pain, swelling and bruising will result, how long I will need to be off work, how long healing will take and whether I will be left with any scars?
- Can I afford it?

If the answer to all these questions is 'yes', then consult your GP to discuss the options, including the possibility of getting help on the NHS. Referral to a cosmetic surgeon should ideally be done by your GP so that all your medical details can be forwarded to him or her.

Because of the cost, cosmetic surgery is available on the NHS only if the surgeon feels there are overriding physical or psychological reasons for doing it. Waiting lists for these operations can be very long. For these reasons, most people opt to have cosmetic surgery done privately.

Cosmetic surgery has few legal safeguards. Anyone can set up a private cosmetic surgery clinic, call him- or herself a consultant, advertise for patients, and even operate, as long as he or she does not pretend to be a doctor. A lot of cosmetic surgery is done in private hospitals and clinics by NHS surgeons, but there are no set minimum training levels, so surgeons from any field can, and do, use skills learned in other operations for cosmetic surgery. There are no guarantees, therefore, that your operation will not be the first of its sort for the surgeon.

If your GP cannot or will not refer you to a cosmetic surgeon or you want to look for one yourself, make sure you check the following details.

- Will the surgeon I met actually do the operation?
- What are his or her qualifications?
- Is he or she a member of BAPS or BAAPS? (See below)
- How many times and how recently has he or she done the operation?
- Does he or she have insurance?

Beware of clinics that ask you to make a decision or even put down a payment before you are allowed to meet a surgeon. Ideally, you should meet a surgeon at your first consultation. He or she should explain the operation and the risks involved, examine you and advise you on your suitability for it. If possible, see two or three surgeons and ask about their experience and qualifications. Choose a surgeon you are comfortable with and avoid one who urges you to have surgery.

Private clinics often proudly advertise that their surgeons are Fellows of the Royal College of Surgeons (FRCS), but this guarantees only that the surgeon has a basic level of surgical training. The British Association of Plastic Surgeons (BAPS)★ and the British Association of Aesthetic Plastic Surgeons (BAAPS)★ are the two professional bodies recognised by the Royal College of Surgeons. The General Medical Council (GMC) has a specialist register with the names of qualified plastic surgeons.

Cosmetic surgery operations considered to be 'major' are those that usually involve the use of a general anaesthetic and some time in hospital. They include face-lifts, nose reshaping, breast surgery and liposuction. 'Minor' cosmetic surgery procedures are those that are done under local anaesthetic – they are not minor in terms of cost, risks or discomfort. They include treatment for broken capillaries ('spiders') and wrinkles, and the removal of tattoos. (See Chapter 9 for more about treatment of these problems.)

Face-lifts

A face-lift can restore a more youthful appearance to a scraggy neck and jowls. It cannot remove the fine lines around the mouth and eyes, and may not affect the grooves between the nose and the mouth. You can get some idea of the final result by pulling up the skin in front of your ears. The operation is most successful for people aged 40–60, because their skin is still elastic.

There are various types of face-lift. Depending on the type of surgery a face-lift could cost between £3,000 and £10,000, and its effects could last up to ten years.

The simplest operation involves making cuts in the facial skin, which is then pulled taut, any excess trimmed off, and the wound re-stitched. In more complex operations, deeper cuts are made and the underlying structures are also pulled upwards and the muscles tightened, creating a more lasting effect. This can be combined with surgery on the eyebrows and lower eyelids to reduce bags under the eyes.

The more drastic the procedure, the greater the risk of extensive swelling and scarring. There is also a danger of damage to facial nerves, resulting in numbness or facial paralysis, although this is usually temporary. Rare side-effects of face-lifts, which may be permanent, include persistent pain in the cheeks or ears, asymmetrical facial expressions owing to muscle weakness, darkened skin in the areas where bruising occurred, the formation of red spider veins on the skin, hair loss over scars, and lumpy, thick scars.

Nose reshaping

Most requests for nose reshaping come from people who think their nose is too big, too long, too hooked or too bumpy. The tip of the nose tends to droop a bit as people age, and surgery to tilt the end up a little is fairly easy to do. As the nose usually continues growing till a person is 20, surgery is not recommended for people below that age.

An operation on the nose can cost between £3,000 and £4,000, and the results generally last forever. The main risk with nose surgery is that you may not like the final result.

The upper third of the nose is a pyramid-shaped piece of bone, the lower two-thirds are softer cartilage, and the tip of the nose is made from two domes of this cartilage. A septum, or wall, runs inside the nose, dividing it in two. For nose reduction, the surgeon moves the nasal bones inwards to make the bridge of the nose narrower. If the tip needs moving upwards, the septum and the cartilage are trimmed to reshape the tip. All the work is usually done from inside the nose, with no need for external cuts. This is called 'closed rhinoplasty'. Sometimes a cut is made in the fleshy part between the nostrils, and this is known as 'open rhinoplasty'. To build up a squashed-looking nose, the surgeon can add cartilage from the ear or a rib, bone from the skull, or silicone implants.

Liposuction

Liposuction is a means to remove unwanted fat. It is not a way to lose weight and should be used only as a last resort after dieting and exercise have been used to get as near as possible to the desired weight. It is most successful for people in their twenties and thirties, as their skin is still stretchy, and is effective on excess fat which will not shift with diet or exercise. Cellulite, which is visible sub-cutaneous fat, cannot be tackled by liposuction.

Liposuction costs between £1,000 and £5,000. The fat may return with weight gain or ageing.

The operation is almost always carried out under general anaesthetic but may not require an overnight hospital stay. The surgeon inserts a fine tube attached to a vacuum pump through the skin and into the fat layer, and moves it around to suck out an even layer of fat. Alternative methods use other ways of breaking up the fat, such as laser, ultrasound or electrical current, but the results and risks are similar.

Bruising, clots under the skin and discomfort are common problems after the surgery. In the longer term, excess skin may look wrinkled and saggy. Persistent swelling and loss of sensation in the skin usually settle down by six months, but occasionally remain a permanent problem. A major risk is that you may be disappointed by the result.

Breast reduction

In this operation, cuts are made around the nipple to reposition it, then down and along the underside of the breast; then the lower part of the breast is removed to make it smaller. Fat in the armpit may also be removed by liposuction (see above). The skin is trimmed, and the scars that form correspond to the cuts.

Breast reduction costs between £3,500 and £4,500. The result is permanent, but changes in weight and age will still affect the size of the breasts.

Risks include blood clots under the skin, which usually drain away but may need to be removed, poor scar healing, damage to the nipple (reducing sensation and the ability to breast-feed), and changes to the nipple colour. Unsightly scars or uneven-sized or -shaped breasts are fairly common risks. Small areas of fat in the breast may die as they are deprived of their blood supply, and this can cause a red, hot area which may drain away or form a lump which can be removed.

Breast enlargement

Breast enlargement, or 'augmentation', is best done on women aged between their late teens and late forties. The surgeon makes a cut in the armpit, around the lower half of the areola (the darker part of the breast surrounding the nipple), or on the underside of the breast. Keyhole surgery allows much smaller cuts to be made. An implant is inserted either just in front of or just behind the muscle of the chest wall. All implants consist of a silicone bag with a filling, which could be soft silicone gel, saline (salt water), soya-bean oil, hydrogel or polyethylene glycol. The operation is always done under general anaesthetic and a one-night stay in hospital is normal.

Breast augmentation costs between £3,000 and £4,000. The life of most implants is between 10 and 15 years.

The most common risk of breast augmentation is a poor cosmetic result, with uneven or lopsided breasts. Blood clots, bruising, infection and pain may all occur, and numbness around the nipple or occasionally increased sensation and tenderness around the nipple are possible risks. Scar tissue will develop around the implants, and the extent of this tissue will determine the final appearance of your breasts. The silicone gel implants can feel hard at first and usually soften up, but for some women they remain hard, lumpy and painful.

There has been a great deal of controversy about the safety of silicone implants. Although most of the scare claims have been refuted, concerns remain that silicone may leak out of the implants and cause auto-immune connective-tissue disorders such as rheumatoid arthritis. A report in July 1998 by the Independent Review Group (IRG) set up by the UK government found no 'conclusive' evidence that women with silicone gel implants are any more likely to have health problems, but that 'there is some risk associated with the use of any implant'. Any woman considering having such implants should discuss this issue with her surgeon before the operation.

Drinking

Q *How do I know whether I am drinking too much? Drinking is part of my work culture. I never feel drunk, and as far as I'm aware I'm not dependent on alcohol – although, to be fair, I never go for more than a day or two without a few drinks.*

A If you are asking this question, you probably are drinking too much. Ask yourself whether, on any single occasion in the last three months, you have had more than five alcoholic drinks. Then ask yourself how many days a week you usually have a drink, and how many units you have each time. A unit of alcohol is equivalent to:

- half a pint (250ml) of average-strength beer
- a glass (125ml) of wine
- a standard measure (25ml) of spirits
- a standard measure of fortified wine such as sherry or port.

In recent years the government's advice on sensible drinking has been for men to drink no more than 21 units, and women no more than 14 units, a week. It is now considered more helpful to think in terms of daily alcohol intake. Men are recommended to drink no more than three to four units a day and women no more than two to three units a day. Men consistently drinking four units a day (and women three) incur a progressive health risk.

The other way to assess your drinking is to ask yourself the 'CAGE' questions:

- Have you ever felt you should **Cut** down on drinking?
- Have people **Annoyed** you by criticising your drinking?
- Have you ever felt **Guilty** about your drinking?
- Have you ever had an **'Eye-opener'** – a drink first thing to steady your nerves?

One 'yes' means you should probably cut down. More than one 'yes' means you may be more dependent than you realise and should seek help.

Q *I am quite a heavy drinker. I don't feel that this is a problem, but recently one or two of my friends have made comments about my drinking habits and behaviour, and even suggested that I should seek help. How do I know if I am an alcoholic and how do I get help if I am?*

A What you need to do first is assess whether you are drinking too much (see previous question), but bear in mind that not everyone who drinks too much is an alcoholic. Being an alcoholic means suffering from alcoholism, which is a physical dependence on alcohol. Typically, someone who is an alcoholic:

- has a very strong urge to drink alcohol
- can drink more and more with less and less effect and hardly ever actually get drunk
- starts to get withdrawal symptoms including feelings of nausea, sweatiness and shaking if he or she cannot get alcohol.

Another sign of alcoholism is drinking in the mornings and to stave off the effects of withdrawal. In the most extreme stages of alcoholism, sufferers may get the 'DTs' (delirium tremens) with memory loss, confusion and shaking hands.

If you think you may be dependent on alcohol, you should get expert help. Start by contacting your GP. He or she can put you in touch with an alcohol dependence clinic (or an alcohol advice centre). You may be given medication, which can help:

- treat underlying problems such as depression
- help reverse some of the ill-effects of the alcohol
- fight the urge to drink
- counteract the unpleasant symptoms of withdrawal
- maintain abstinence once you have given up drinking.

Alcoholics Anonymous (AA)* offers group therapy in structured weekly meetings with a group of people with a similar problem, and can provide very useful support. Many alcoholics attend AA meetings long after they have recovered. Families and friends of alcoholics are often put under a great deal of strain and their needs and concerns also need to be recognised. Al-Anon Family Groups UK* is an organisation that could provide them with support.

Counselling to address the underlying reasons for a person's alcoholism and to help recovery is also useful.

Smoking

Q *I am desperate to give up smoking and have tried all the products on offer several times. The longest time I have managed is nine months, two years ago. Can you suggest anything that might help me succeed?*

A Giving up smoking is hard and it is admirable that you keep try-ing. Anyone with any interest in their health must want to quit because it is the single biggest preventable cause of disease (cancers, heart attacks and strokes – see boxes later in this chapter) and pre-mature death. Tobacco smoking causes at least 20 per cent of all deaths in the UK, and about half of all regular smokers will eventu-ally be killed by their habit. Fewer than 10 per cent of lung cancer patients survive more than five years after diagnosis. In addition to cancers and heart disease, smoking causes a wide range of other health problems: for example, in women it can lead to an earlier menopause, and in men, it has been associated with sperm abnor-malities and impotence. More than 17,000 children are admitted to hospital every year because of the effects of passive smoking.

Nicotine replacement therapy (NRT) really does work, and is now available on the NHS. Using the patches probably gives the best long-term chance of quitting. Other forms of NRT include gum, tablets, inhalers and nasal sprays. Some counselling and sup-port (from your GP, practice nurse or specialist smoking cessation clinic) is also helpful in addition to using NRT.

The drug bupropion (Zyban) has provided a very welcome boost to smokers trying to quit. Developed initially as an antidepressant, Zyban is a tablet, available on the NHS. You start taking a daily tablet one week before quitting smoking. The total length of the course is two months and many people use NRT at the same time. The chief side-effect of Zyban is sleep disturbance, with many users reporting that they are unable to sleep through the night or get off to sleep. Some people also find that it causes a dry mouth. Your GP will be able to let you know whether Zyban is suitable for you, as it should not be prescribed to some people – for example, those who have, or have had, epilepsy.

Further advice about giving up smoking is available from Action on Smoking and Health (ASH).★

Q *I enjoy a cigar, but my wife is worried that it is an unhealthy habit. I always thought cigars were much safer than cigarettes. Aren't they?*

A Your wife is right. Tobacco smoke from cigars is chemically similar to cigarette smoke and puts you at increased risk of heart disease and lung cancer. Yours is a widely held belief – statistics from the USA show that the number of cigar smokers there rose by 50 per cent between 1998 and 2001, as people increasingly gave up cigarettes. But a recent study of 120,000 US men over the age of 30 showed that current cigar smokers had an increased risk of heart disease compared with non-cigar smokers. The good news is that if you quit, your risk of heart disease quickly returns to that of a non-smoker.

Drugs

Q *I am terribly worried that my 15-year-old son may be taking drugs. He has a new group of friends who are much older than him, and I have no idea what he gets up to when he is out in the evenings. I suppose I may be over-reacting, but I don't know anything about drugs or how serious the dangers are. What should I do?*

A Young people today are undoubtedly more likely to be exposed to illicit drugs than their parents were, and as a parent you cannot ignore the possibility that your child may come into contact with drugs as he or she is growing up. According to the 1999 European school survey project on alcohol and other drugs, 35 per cent of 15- to 16-year-olds in the UK had used cannabis in that year, and 12 per cent had used other illicit drugs apart from cannabis.

Social and peer group influences play a large part in a young person's decision to experiment with drugs. It would probably help if you are able to meet and get to know your son's friends, and try to maintain good communication with him so you can help him respond sensibly to their influences. One appeal of these drugs is, of course, that they have pleasurable effects – something which may be ignored by educationalists and parents.

It can be difficult to tell whether your teenager is taking drugs because often the warning signs are also perfectly normal features of adolescence! It may sometimes be hard to believe that the parents of children who have become involved with drugs did not notice that anything was wrong – but teenagers can be moody and unpredictable for reasons of their own. That said, the following could be warning signs of someone taking drugs: mood changes that are out of character or are sudden; unusual sleep patterns (e.g. lying in bed all day or pacing around at night); evasive answers or secretive behaviour. Additional signs are discovering that money is going missing or that your son is selling some of his belongings, or finding rubbish that is unusual, such as tablets, needles, bits of foil, things that smell of glue, etc.

If you notice any of these signs try not to jump to conclusions. Talk to your son in as open and non-confrontational a way as possible. If you feel you need to talk to his teachers and friends, be aware that doing this without his consent may alienate him. You can inform yourself by contacting the National Drugs Helpline.★ This offers confidential counselling, advice and information from sympathetic and fully trained staff, and the number will not appear on any itemised phone bills. Other support organisations and helplines are Parents Against Drug Abuse★ and Release.★ Ask your GP for help in accessing specialist services if need be. You may need to share your concerns and stresses with a counsellor, and your GP should be able to point you in the right direction.

The Health Education Board for Scotland★ has a very informative web site on the effects and relative risks of the main illicit drugs available in the UK.

Q *I suffer from osteoarthritis. Sometimes the pain is so bad that I feel I would be willing to try anything. I have heard that cannabis can be very good for pain relief. Is this true?*

A There are many accounts of people with conditions such as multiple sclerosis (MS – see page 30) using cannabis for relief of pain, as well as other symptoms of the condition. No definitive clinical evidence yet exists to prove that it is beneficial. Two major trials have been funded by the Medical Research Council, which will evaluate cannabis (given in tablet form to MS sufferers) for its effectiveness in pain relief. Results should be available by 2003. At the moment, cannabis cannot be prescribed by doctors in the UK and is used legally only within these clinical trials. Its use for any other purpose is still strictly illegal, although courts have tended to be lenient on people found in possession of cannabis for medicinal purposes. The long-term safety of the drug has not yet been properly evaluated.

Tiredness and debility

Q *Recently I have been feeling constantly tired. I sleep soundly, wake up OK, but as the day progresses I get more and more tired. By midday I am ready to sleep and do sleep if I am at home. I am also very thirsty and out of breath. There is a history of high blood pressure and diabetes in the family. Could I be suffering from either of these?*

A Thirst and tiredness can certainly be signs of diabetes, and with your family history you should have a urine or blood test to check for it. Shortness of breath may be a sign of anaemia: you can have a blood test for this. It may also be linked to high blood pressure.

You sound as though you could do with a full health MOT, including measurement of weight and blood pressure, examination of your heart and lungs, a chest X-ray and blood tests for anaemia, thyroid, kidney function and sugar. An ECG (electrocardiogram) to check your heart would also be a good idea. Your GP should be able to do or arrange for all these tests, if he or she thinks they are appropriate. You may well find that there is no specific underlying problem – often, in fact, no physical cause is found. Shortness of breath and tiredness can also reflect being overweight and not doing enough (or any) exercise. But certainly you need to have a check-up before leaping to any conclusions.

(For more about diabetes, high blood pressure and thyroid problems, see boxes earlier in this chapter.)

Anaemia

'Anaemia' refers to low haemoglobin – the compound in blood that carries oxygen to the cells. It results from many different conditions, most commonly blood loss, for example after a very heavy period, an operation or an injury. Anaemia can also be caused by vitamin deficiencies, namely folate and B12. Long-standing diseases including rheumatoid arthritis and many cancers can also result in anaemia. Symptoms include breathlessness and tiredness.

ME

Q *I have been ill for over a year and have had a number of tests, which have failed to identify the cause. The doctor's conclusion is that I have ME. Can you tell me more about it, and whether you think there is anything else that could be the cause of my illness?*

A ME (myalgic encephalomyelitis) or CFS (chronic fatigue syndrome), as it is also known, is a great concern for sufferers and for doctors. Its cause remains uncertain, its diagnosis can be tricky and the best treatment options have yet to be proved. And of course if you are suffering from debilitating fatigue, muscle pains and tender glands, it can ruin your life. The criteria for diagnosis set out by the US Centers for Disease Control (CDC) have helped, although there is still no one diagnostic test that proves whether or not you have ME. The CDC states that to have ME you must have four or more of the following symptoms persisting or recurring over six months following the onset of abnormal fatigue:

• loss of your normal level of concentration or short-term memory to an extent that impairs your normal functioning, e.g. at work
• sore throat
• tender glands in the neck or armpits
• headaches of a type that is new for you
• muscle pains
• joint pains in several joints with no signs of redness or swelling of the joints
• unrefreshing sleep
• feeling ill for more than 24 hours after exertion.

Your GP will want to run blood tests to check you do not have anaemia, diabetes, underactive thyroid (see boxes earlier in this chapter) or a current viral illness. Depending on your specific symptoms, you may be referred to a neurologist to specifically rule out multiple sclerosis (MS – see below), as the symptoms of MS and ME may initially be similar.

The ME Association* has a list of consultants who are particularly interested in and sympathetic to ME sufferers, and you could ask your GP to refer you to the most local one for a treatment package that ideally will deal with all aspects of your condition, physical and psychological, and offer help with graded activity, nutrition, occupational therapy and sometimes drug or psychological treatments also.

Multiple sclerosis

Multiple sclerosis (MS) is caused by damage to the protective coating around the nerves in the brain and/or spinal cord. It can occur in sudden episodes, with recovery between attacks, or it can cause ongoing deterioration. Some people with MS suffer only one attack. MS may cause numbness in a limb or in half the body, weakness in the legs, pain in one eye with temporary dim vision, double vision, vertigo, incontinence, difficulty in speaking clearly, mood changes and memory loss, or tremor. It is made worse by exertion and heat. Diagnosis can be difficult.

At present there is no cure for MS. Treatments include supplementing the diet with polyunsaturated fats, using steroids for eye problems, and interferon beta (Betaferon) – a drug that acts by boosting the body's immune system and seems to prevent recurrences.

Lupus

Q *I get very tired, breathless and fed-up. A few years ago I was told I had lupus. How much of what I am feeling is likely to be due to that, and do you have any advice about how to cope with it?*

A Lupus is an auto-immune condition in which the body reacts against itself. It tends to cause joint pains, stiffness, mood changes, hair loss, skin rashes which are precipitated by sunlight, mouth ulcers, tiredness, and in some cases blood clots in the lung and recurrent miscarriages. Inflammation of the kidneys, heart and lungs can also flare up and it is the latter two that can cause breathlessness. There is no overall cure, although the condition tends to wax and wane and can sometimes seemingly disappear for good. Drugs that control inflammation, such as chloroquine (Avloclor), azathioprine (Imuran) and steroids, are used in severe flare-ups. The organisation Lupus UK★ can provide further information.

You need to make sure that you are not anaemic (see page 28), which can cause breathlessness and excessive tiredness. Anaemia could be linked to the lupus, or it may not: it can happen to anyone who has lost lots of blood for whatever reason. For tiredness associated with a flare-up of lupus, you will need to try graded exercise:

pace yourself by trying to do a bit more each day but without getting overtired. A medication review is also a good idea.

You should always seek medical advice for severe and sudden breathlessness, because of the rare cases of blood clots in the lung (pulmonary embolus) or inflammation of the lung, which require urgent treatment.

Insomnia

Q *For years now, on and off, I have had awful trouble sleeping. If I fall asleep I usually sleep all night, but often I simply cannot get to sleep. Many nights I lie awake until the early hours. This can happen for three nights in a row in any one week and I get totally exhausted. Can you suggest anything at all that might help?*

A A lot of people worry a great deal about their sleep patterns – too little, too much, too patchy, too light, too deep. The acid test is whether you wake feeling refreshed and have enough energy during the day to achieve what you want to – and it sounds as though you have a problem because you feel tired during the day. It can be useful to see a counsellor or your GP or practice nurse to talk through some of the issues which may be undermining your sleep. There are some basic questions to ask yourself and simple steps you can try.

- Do you have a wind-down routine before going to sleep? This can include setting a bedtime, avoiding work for two hours beforehand, having a soothing, non-alcoholic and decaffeinated drink, taking a hot bath, and reading a relaxing book or listening to peaceful music.
- Are you physically tired enough to sleep? You may need to do more aerobic, outdoor activity during the day.
- Are you depressed or anxious? Both conditions affect your ability to sleep. See a health professional if you have lost your enjoyment of life, cannot eat, feel tearful and sad, or anxious, panicky and agitated. (See Chapter 2 for more about depression and anxiety.)
- Are the conditions right for you to get to sleep? For example, do you need a better pillow, mattress or duvet? Do you have children sharing your bed and kneeing you in the back all night? Does your partner snore?
- If you cannot sleep, get up and do something soothing – for example, read or have a milky drink. Then go back to bed telling

yourself that you will be able to sleep now but it does not matter if you cannot. The more you fret about not sleeping, the less likely you are to nod off.

- Remedies to help you sleep include homeopathic, herbal, over-the-counter and prescribed drugs. None is a substitute for working out why you cannot sleep and addressing it, but drugs can be useful for a few days to help break the cycle of sleeplessness – although they may become less effective after repeated use. You may prefer to try valerian herbal remedy.

Preventing and detecting disease

Taking aspirin

Q *I am a 62-year-old woman with no particular medical problems. All my friends seem to be taking a junior aspirin a day in the belief that it will fend off strokes and heart attacks. Should I be taking these?*

A The reason for taking aspirin as a prophylactic is that it thins the blood. It is true that if 1,000 healthy people with normal blood pressure were to take aspirin every day for a year, two or three fewer of them would have a non-fatal heart attack or stroke than if they did not take aspirin. However, many of them would also get indigestion or even stomach ulcers as a result, so the benefits do not always outweigh the risks. Aspirin can also exacerbate asthma and cause easy bruising and prolonged bleeding, so cuts and nose bleeds take longer to staunch. People with high blood pressure (see box earlier in this chapter) may be tempted to take aspirin to stave off strokes. But in fact a recent Medical Research Council trial suggested that those with high blood pressure do not get significant protection from the aspirin – far better to take measures to control the blood pressure. So, to ward off strokes and heart attacks get your blood pressure and cholesterol checked, but do not feel you have to copy your friends by taking aspirin.

Self-testing kits

Q *I have seen various home testing kits and machines for sale in our local chemist. My father had bowel cancer and I worry about getting it myself. Is it a good idea to use one of these kits to pick up any warning signs? Are they reliable?*

A There are, as you say, a burgeoning number of self-testing kits now available. Some are very reliable and easy to use, such as the home pregnancy tests, which are based on the same test that is used in hospital laboratories. The chance of inaccuracies with these is very small indeed.

If you have diabetes it is important to monitor your own condition, so kits that allow you to measure your blood glucose levels are valuable. The kits or machines must be checked against laboratory gold standards, which you should be able to organise through your diabetes specialist at the hospital. Your GP will be able to do a blood test to confirm the self-monitoring test.

Likewise, if you have high blood pressure you may find it reassuring to be able to measure it yourself – especially when starting new medication. Or you may want to keep a close eye on your blood pressure if it has been high in the past. It is a good idea to check your machine against your doctor's and also to liaise closely with your doctor to agree a plan of action.

Other tests may be reliable in the results they give, but only provide a small piece of a larger jigsaw. For instance, a self-testing kit for cholesterol will usually give you a reasonably accurate reading. But the correct interpretation of the result will depend on numerous factors, including whether you are at increased risk of heart disease because of your family history, age, smoking or high blood pressure. An isolated cholesterol-level reading is not very useful.

As for bowel cancer, it is worth being tested if you are over 50. Before that age, you are at low risk unless one or more members of your close family have developed bowel cancer at a young age. It is quite likely that we will soon see a national screening programme based on testing for blood in the stool, in 50–69-year-olds, and it is thought that by testing this age group every two years the bowel cancer death rate could be reduced by 20 per cent. The kits available in some pharmacies can be tricky to use and may give unreliable results, so if you think you are at risk it would be worth going to your GP to discuss your concerns rather than relying on a home test. The GP can arrange to have your stool sample tested. One advantage of going to your doctor is that if you do get a positive test result, there is some provision for back-up advice and counselling. If your GP thinks you are at high risk of bowel cancer, you may be advised to be seen at a specialist unit in the hospital.

Heart disease and strokes

High blood pressure, which is the result of narrowed blood vessels, causes further damage to these blood vessels and restricts circulation. Narrowing of the coronary arteries that supply the heart itself can result in the chest pain known as angina. A **heart attack**, or myocardial infarction (MI), occurs when a coronary artery becomes completely blocked and the section of heart muscle which depends on that coronary artery dies. Symptoms of a heart attack may include crushing pain across the chest, pain spreading into the neck, jaw, shoulders or arms; nausea, dizziness and breathlessness. Anyone suspected of having a heart attack should be seen by a doctor as soon as possible.

Heart failure is a syndrome causing fluid retention, shortness of breath on exertion or lying flat, and oedema (swelling), usually most noticeable in the ankles. It may arise as a complication of many different heart diseases.

A **stroke** is caused when a blood vessel in the brain becomes blocked, and the part of the brain dependent on that blood vessel is severely damaged. The part of the body controlled by the affected part of the brain is unable to function. Over a few hours, one side of the body feels like a dead weight, hangs limply and then becomes rigid and numb. Vision may be impaired and it may be difficult to speak coherently. Severe strokes can cause total paralysis.

Heart disease and strokes are the biggest cause of death in the UK. The risk of these diseases increases as you get older and is higher if you have a family history of heart disease and strokes. Obviously these factors are beyond your control, but there are other ways that you can minimise the risk.

Smoking is a major cause of damage to blood vessels in the heart, brain or general circulation. Stopping smoking, controlling high blood pressure, keeping to a low-fat diet, avoiding excess alcohol consumption, treating high blood cholesterol levels and taking regular exercise are the best ways to prevent heart attacks, strokes and other forms of damage to the heart and circulation.

A new test likely to reach our high-street chemists soon is a blood test known as DR-70tm (tumour marker), which is already on sale in Canada and China. The claim is that it can detect 13 different cancers, including common ones such as lung, bowel, ovarian and stomach cancer. This is based on the notion that cancer cells release chemicals known as proteases, which can be measured in the blood. However, the reliability of this test is not proven.

Vaccinations

Q *I would like to take my child to a homeopath instead of a GP because I am worried about vaccinations and conventional medications like antibiotics that I believe can damage a small child's natural immunity. What do you think?*

A It does not necessarily need to be an 'either/or' situation. Many people consult their GPs regularly but also see a homeopath or other complementary health practitioner from time to time. There is rarely any inherent contradiction, and sometimes the views, therapies and advice offered by two different practitioners can be valuable, particularly when dealing with tricky problems such as childhood eczema and asthma.

A degree of scepticism about conventional and complementary therapies alike is healthy – it is useful to know whether evidence exists to support a treatment. There are certain interventions in conventional medicine (e.g. antibiotics for sore throats, grommets for glue ear) which are not supported by good evidence, and some aspects of complementary therapies also lack convincing evidence. Naturally we are also guided in our choice of therapies by confidence in the practitioner, recommendations by friends and family and our own experience of what has worked for us.

One of the key attractions of homeopathy is that it is extremely safe and preparations can be given to children and pregnant women. The philosophy of restoring the body's natural balance using very dilute preparations is attractive to many. Trials are not universally encouraging, but much research remains to be done. However, homeopathic 'immunisation' offers no protection against infectious diseases, and many homeopaths do encourage routine childhood vaccinations.

Immunisation helps the body develop lasting resistance to serious and often fatal infections and diseases, and has saved hundreds of thousands of children from death and handicap. Since the introduction of routine childhood immunisation, many diseases including poliomyelitis, tetanus and diphtheria have been virtually eliminated.

Critics of immunisation say that the child's body is not allowed to develop natural immunity, that immunity produced after injections may not be as long-lasting as that which is produced naturally, and that side-effects ranging from rare but serious neurological damage such as fits, to more common and 'minor' side-effects such as fever and pain at the injection site, are high prices to pay for protection from illnesses, some of which are not very dangerous in themselves.

Advocates of routine immunisation programmes counter that serious side-effects such as neurological damage are very rare indeed and are far outweighed by the risk of neurological damage from the disease itself. The minor side-effects of vaccination are milder than even the mildest case of the illness itself. There is no good evidence that immunisation weakens the immune system; indeed it may stimulate it, and the immune system still fights all the viruses and other bugs against which a person is not immunised. To rely on natural immunity against the illnesses which most children are vaccinated against is potentially dangerous, as a child is unlikely to encounter those illnesses in childhood and will not have the opportunity to build up any resistance against infections such as meningitis, for example.

Girls who are not immunised against rubella (German measles) may contract it when pregnant, with potentially dangerous implications for the unborn child. Boys who are not immunised against rubella can contract it in adulthood and pass it on to non-immune pregnant women. Mumps in adolescence or adulthood can affect male fertility, and measles and meningitis are potentially fatal illnesses.

Immunisation gives the child a 'mini dose' of an infection, and his or her immune system then builds resistance to the infection from this tiny dose. The programme begins at the age of two months. The first vaccines given are triple antigen (to protect against diphtheria, whooping cough and tetanus), Hib vaccine (to protect against meningitis), meningitis C and poliomyelitis vaccine. At the age of one year, the MMR vaccine is given to protect against measles, mumps and rubella.

Minor side-effects such as redness or soreness at the site of the injection are common. These may last a day or two. Fever sometimes occurs and may be relieved by giving your child an appropriate dose of paracetamol mixture for his or her age. Serious side-effects are exceedingly rare and are most unlikely to cause any permanent harm to your child. However, you should contact your doctor immediately if your child:

- has a high fever (38°C or more)
- is very irritable or sleepy
- has any other unexplained problems.

Babies can be immunised safely if they have minor coughs or colds without a fever, or if they are taking antibiotics but are well. Children with asthma, eczema, hay fever and allergies may be safely immunised but remember to tell your GP if your child has had a severe allergic reaction to egg. Talk to your GP again before the measles vaccine is given at the age of one year.
(See Chapter 3 for autism and the MMR, and Chapter 11 for more information on the MMR and also meningitis C vaccinations.)

Cancer

Q *There has been a lot of cancer in my family, and I worry about whether I am at risk. Would it be worth asking my GP for a referral to a specialist?*

A Your concern is understandable, but do not forget that there is a lot we can do to reduce the risk of cancer (see below), and that although there is much we still do not know about the genetics of cancers, most are not linked and are probably not inherited. You should certainly ask to be referred if you have a close relative who was under 40 when diagnosed with a common cancer, such as breast, ovarian, bowel, stomach or prostate cancer, or if you have two close relatives with any of those cancers diagnosed under the age of 50. Even if you do not fall into those categories, but you are concerned, you could ask to be referred to a genetics clinic. Before you go, if possible try to glean as much information as you can from relatives, as to who had what and at what ages they were diagnosed.

Cancer

Cancer is a disease of the body's cells. Normally, all cells divide and reproduce themselves in an orderly and controlled manner. Cancerous cells, however, multiply without proper control, forming a lump (tumour) or a collection of abnormal cells, as in the case of leukaemia.

Sometimes cancer cells break away from a tumour and travel to other parts of the body via the bloodstream or lymphatic system. The lymphatic system is a network of fine channels that run throughout the body and are part of the body's protection against infection and cancer. When the cancer cells reach other parts of the body they may settle and start to develop into new tumours. (See relevant chapters in this book for more about cancers in particular parts of the body.)

Further information and advice is available from organisations such as the Cancer Research Campaign.*

Prevention

Cancer is the second biggest killer in the UK, after heart disease and strokes. At least 50 per cent of cancers are strongly related to lifestyle, and therefore could be prevented. You can minimise the risk by observing some common-sense guidelines:

- do not smoke, moderate your alcohol intake, eat healthily and exercise regularly
- avoid excessive exposure to the sun and protect your skin with sun cream, light clothing and a hat
- follow health and safety instructions relating to the production or handling of any substance that may cause cancer
- see a doctor if you notice a lump or any change in a mole, or have any abnormal bleeding
- see a doctor if you have problems that persist, such as a cough, hoarseness, a change in bowel habits or unexplained weight loss
- for women, have a cervical smear test regularly and check your breasts regularly; undergo mammography regularly if you are over 50.

Treatment

Surgery is usually performed to remove any lump. This may be followed by chemotherapy or radiotherapy.

Chemotherapy drugs work by interfering with the ability of a cancer cell to divide and reproduce itself. The affected cells become damaged and eventually die. As the drugs are carried in the blood, they can reach cancer cells all over the body. Unfortunately, chemotherapy drugs can also affect normal cells in your body, sometimes causing unpleasant side-effects. Normal cells, however, quickly regrow, so any damage to them is usually temporary and most side-effects will disappear after treatment. Chemotherapy can, however, have an effect on fertility, and you should discuss any concerns about this with your doctor.

Radiotherapy uses X-rays to destroy the tumour. Although there is concern about the dangers of radiation, when used properly the risks are small and are greatly outweighed by the benefits. Radiotherapy may be given before or after surgery, and may also be given in lower doses to relieve symptoms of the disease, for example, to lessen pain. This is called palliative treatment.

Total body irradiation is a form of radiotherapy often given to patients who are having a bone marrow transplant, for example for leukaemia. A large single dose (or six to eight smaller doses) of radiation is given to the whole body to destroy the cells of the bone marrow. The new bone marrow, either from a donor or taken from the patient before his or her irradiation, then takes its place.

Some **drugs**, such as interferon (Roferon), are currently being used in the treatment of cancers, and many others are presently undergoing trials. Interferon boosts the body's immune response to help it fight off the invading cancer cells. Hormonal treatments, such as goserelin (Zoladex), are used in prostate cancer. Vaccines against cancers such as melanoma are being worked on, and there is hope for the future use of gene therapy in the detection and even cure of a range of cancers.

Q *I have just been diagnosed as having breast cancer. I feel shocked and frightened about the cancer, but also very unhappy about the treatment being offered – a course of chemotherapy followed by radiotherapy. I would be happier with some sort of alternative therapy, although to be honest I am quite confused by it all. Can you offer any guidance?*

A It is of course a terrible shock to learn that you have breast cancer. You may be catapulted from being a normally healthy person, often with little contact with doctors, into the arms of the medical profession. You may not even feel ill; just overwhelmed by the diagnosis and frightened about the future and the impact of treatment. It is natural to reject therapeutic options offered to you and to shop around for alternatives, to inform yourself widely and seek second opinions. Conventional and complementary therapies are often compatible: for example, reflexology and radiotherapy can happily coexist. Ultimately, however, you have to come off the fence and either accept or reject the treatment being offered. In many women's experiences, their worst nightmares do not materialise and the treatment programmes are often less traumatic than they fear. Most of us have a strong instinct for survival and if we are offered treatment, we take it even if it makes us feel sick and tired for a few weeks.

A number of different types of treatment are available to people with cancer. Further advice and information is available from CancerBACUP.★

- **Conventional** therapies are the treatments used within mainstream medicine. For the treatment of cancer these consist of surgery, radiotherapy, chemotherapy and hormone treatment (see box above). All these treatments have usually been tested in clinical trials and through long experience with patients.
- **Complementary** therapies, in the strictest sense of the term, are those treatments which are used in conjunction with the conventional treatments. Examples include massage and reflexology. Some complementary therapies may be available through the NHS. However, the complementary medicine industry itself generally uses the term to include 'alternative' therapies.
- **Alternative** therapies, in the strictest sense, are those treatments which are intended to be used instead of conventional treatments. Examples include acupuncture and homeopathy.

Certain complementary therapies, such as counselling and physio-therapy, are now regarded as standard medical practice, and in many cancer centres counselling is available as part of the treatment. Other complementary therapies, such as relaxation and massage, while not part of conventional treatment, are accepted by doctors because they can help people feel better and cope better with their illness, and also they tend to cause no harm. These too are available in many cancer centres. Studies of some complementary therapies, such as certain types of psychotherapy, relaxation and hypnotherapy, have shown an improvement in patients' quality of life. Several studies to evaluate other complementary therapies, such as aroma-therapy, are now in progress and will help to determine whether there are real benefits.

Some alternative therapies have caused a conflict of views between doctors and alternative practitioners. Most of these treat-ments have never been scientifically studied or validated, and doc-tors are concerned that certain therapies may give patients false hope and occasionally may even be harmful, and that patients may turn away from conventional treatments that could help them. People with cancer can be very vulnerable and there have been cases when people have been misled by promises of a miracle cure.

If you are considering using complementary or alternative thera-pies talk to your doctor for advice and support. Doctors are gener-ally supportive of patients using any complementary therapies which help them cope better with their illness. Sometimes people who seek alternatives to conventional treatments do so because they are confused, lack information, or feel they have not been given enough time to ask questions or talk about their concerns. This can lead to misunderstandings about their treatment, or they may feel there is nothing more their doctor can do for them. It is important to get all the information you need from your doctor. Take a friend or relative with you for support and write down a list of your most important questions beforehand.

If you are considering complementary therapies the following suggestions may help you.

- Always use a qualified therapist who belongs to a professional body. The organisations listed at the back of this book can give you names of registered therapists and advice on what to look for.

- Check the cost of treatment beforehand to make sure you are being fairly charged. Again, the organisations listed at the back of this book should be able to give you an idea of what is usual.
- Talk the matter over with your doctor or nurse and ask for their advice, especially if you are going to have a therapy which involves taking pills or medicines.
- Ask your doctor or nurse if complementary therapies are available at your treatment hospital, or through your GP's practice, or if they can recommend any therapies or practitioners.
- Choose the complementary therapy that suits your individual needs. If you are not sure and would like to know what other patients have found helpful, contact a patient support group. Support groups often offer complementary therapies.
- Do not be misled by promises of cures. For example, no reputable therapist would claim to be able to cure cancer.

More information can be found in *The Which? Guide to Complementary Medicine*.

Chapter 2

Psychological concerns and the nervous system

Although we may find it relatively easy to discuss physical problems with our families, friends or a doctor, admitting to psychological distress is harder. People who would not normally tolerate being in physical pain for any length of time will often put up with being depressed or anxious for years. Some who grew up in Britain during the Second World War, for example, harbour a feeling that depression is self-indulgent, and that asking for help is an admission of failure. However, our modern Western culture boasts a high proportion of sufferers from depression, stress or anxiety. Irrational fears, phobias, obsessions or difficulty with social situations are also not uncommon. Medical and psychotherapeutic expertise is available to deal with all these problems, and the relief of finding a solution is well worth the effort it may take to seek help.

The spectrum of psychological illnesses is comparable to that of physical illnesses. Despite this, mental illness is still feared in our society and carries a stigma. Nowadays there are effective drugs to control the symptoms of diseases such as schizophrenia and manic depression, and it is a tragedy that anyone suffering from such an illness should miss out on treatment because of ignorance.

Conditions that make people disturbed or unable to interact normally with others, such as autism, Asperger's syndrome or Tourette's syndrome, need to be identified as soon as possible to help the individual and carers to cope. Diagnostic labels are obviously not a cure in themselves, but they do open the door to understanding a sufferer's behaviour and to accessing appropriate help.

This chapter covers all these conditions. It also offers advice on dealing with the psychological damage resulting from sexual abuse.

In addition it looks at premenstrual syndrome, post-natal depression, eating disorders, memory loss, and conditions of the nervous system such as stammering. Whatever your concern, the information provided should aid your understanding and give you the confidence and courage to seek help.

Further advice and support is available from a number of support organisations, listed at the back of the book. MIND,* which aims to help those in mental distress and campaigns for better services and resources for the mentally distressed, is the leading mental health charity in England and Wales. The organisation SANE* has a national mental health helpline, Saneline.

Talking therapies

All 'talking therapies' or types of counselling share certain characteristics – they involve you, the client, talking to a therapist to explore problems you are having – but your experience of them will depend on your personality and current state of mind, as well as the therapist's character, training and approach. Talking therapies work by allowing you to share problems, understand your state of mind better and work towards resolving troubling issues. The therapist may suggest that you do certain tasks, make lists of your problems or find novel ways of looking at old problems, or may seem to just bounce back your words to you. You may notice positive changes within a couple of sessions; generally, though, you may require many sessions over long periods. Talking therapies are not a panacea; they work for some people some of the time but would never claim to 'cure' every ill.

Psychodynamic psychotherapy This involves exploring the feelings clients have for others, especially family members. You may need to delve into past relationships and experiences to try to understand how they affect your current feelings. Some people find this process painful and disruptive. Other ways of exploring the sub-conscious, including the interpretation of dreams, may also be used.

Behavioural therapy In this type of therapy, there is less emphasis on delving into the past and far more on modifying undesirable behaviour. A specific problem is identified and a programme to overcome it

---

Depression

Q *I seem to suffer from recurring depression. How can I tell and what can I do about it?*

A We all feel fed up and down at times, but clinical depression is different; it is a debilitating illness that interferes with normal life and stops us functioning adequately. Depression does not just affect your mood, it stops you enjoying life in any way. There is much better recognition and treatment of depression than there used to be; however, the condition remains underdiagnosed by doctors and undetected in many people, especially those who find it hard to

---

is worked out. The programme is broken down into a series of tasks to be achieved. You may be asked to keep a detailed diary to chart progress. You will be taught skills, which will then be reinforced (e.g. if you have a phobia about closed spaces you will be gradually introduced to using a lift or travelling on the Tube). You will also be taught techniques and exercises to control anxiety. Clients tend to respond rapidly to treatment but their underlying psychological problems may not be identified or tackled. Behavioural therapy works particularly well for phobias, panic attacks, some sexual problems and obsessive-compulsive disorders.

Cognitive behavioural therapy (CBT) CBT tries to change the way clients think, behave and view the world. You may be advised to keep a diary of situations, moods and thoughts; the therapist could use that to point out distorted ways of thinking and how they can be changed. CBT is particularly good for phobias, and panic and anxiety attacks. It can help depression, obsessive-compulsive disorders and bulimia.

Family and marital therapy This involves all members of a family or the marital partners seeing the therapist together, and could use any of the counselling techniques described above. Individuals may also continue to have counselling on their own but the warring couple of a disturbed family is seen as a unit, with the therapist available to facilitate the discussion of problems, set boundaries and help to find a way forward, or to manage change if marital breakdown becomes inevitable.

express their emotions. The following symptoms are indicators of depression:

- lack of energy
- no enjoyment or sense of excitement about anything
- lack of self-confidence – feeling useless, inadequate and hopeless
- finding it hard to make even simple decisions
- feeling negative, sad, tired and tearful
- sleep disturbance – often waking in the early hours of the morning
- appetite disturbance – often not wanting to eat but sometimes overeating; weight loss
- sexual disturbance – no interest in sex
- suicidal thoughts.

Some people have a depressive personality and are prone to a negative way of thinking. This may be an inherited tendency or reinforced by behaviour learned in childhood. Many of us become depressed after a series of unhappy events, such as bereavement, divorce or redundancy. Sometimes a series of stressful events, such as moving house, changing jobs or the children leaving home, can pile up and become overwhelming. Often depression seemingly comes out of the blue and envelops us.

In the vast majority of cases, whatever the cause, we recover from depression. It can be seen as going into a tunnel – it is dark, lonely and we have no idea why we are in it – but usually, without warning, the light appears and we gradually exit from the tunnel feeling psychologically battered but better.

Medication can alleviate depression. Newer antidepressants are specifically geared towards improving the concentration of chemical messengers that carry signals between nerves in the brain. The best known is fluoxetine (Prozac – see below), but there are many products on the market, which your GP will be able to advise you about. Herbal treatments include St John's wort, which is proven to be helpful in cases of mild to moderate depression but is not without potential side-effects.

'Talking therapies' can also be very helpful; counsellors may be associated with your GP's surgery, referred to by a psychiatrist or recommended by friends or mental health organisations such as MIND.★ Therapists vary in their approach and obviously you need to find one to whom you can relate. Cognitive behavioural therapy (CBT) takes a problem-solving approach – one which many find particularly useful.

Support is also available from the Samaritans★ and groups such as the Depression Alliance.★

Q *I've been a bit depressed off and on for the past two years. My GP is always trying to get me to go for counselling but I'm very sceptical. Does it actually work any better than talking to a friend over a cup of tea?*

A Counselling within general practice has become very widespread and most people like it and say that they feel better for it. This does not mean that it is a panacea – success obviously depends on how depressed you are and why, the skill of the counsellor and your own attitude to counselling. The vast majority of people with mild depression, such as yourself, get better whether they have treatment or not. There is some evidence that seeing a practice-based counsellor for the usual eight sessions or fewer helps people to recover more than does GP care alone. Counselling also seems to result in fewer referrals to psychiatrists, less prescribing of anti-depressant drugs, and greater levels of satisfaction by clients. So it probably does help, but you still should not go in for it if you do not want to.

Q *I have a close friend who is prone to bouts of fairly severe depression. When his business or personal life becomes stressful, he is overcome by black thoughts, feels hopeless and can't see his way out of the situation. I feel worried and powerless to help him when he's in this state. What should I do?*

A It is often difficult to know what to say to someone who is very depressed – it may seem that you cannot say anything right, because everything is interpreted in a very negative way. (Cognitive behavioural therapy is particularly effective in such cases because it helps people with those negative thoughts.) It can be very difficult to know what depressed people want – because often these people themselves do not know what they want. They may be very withdrawn and irritable but at the same time unable to do without your help and support. They may be very worried but unwilling or unable to accept advice. So try to be as patient and understanding as possible.

Practical help may be easier to offer and is very valuable. Make sure that your friend is able to look after himself properly. If you find that he is seriously neglecting himself by not eating or drinking, seek medical help immediately. If he talks of self-harm or suicide, this should be taken seriously and professional help should be obtained.

It is also important that you give yourself the space and time you need to recharge your batteries. Make sure that you are able to spend some time on your own or with trusted friends who will give you the support you need at this time. If your friend has to go into hospital, make sure that you share the visiting with someone else. You will be better able to support him if you yourself have had some time to rest.

Antidepressants

Q *I have been very depressed recently and my GP has prescribed Prozac. However, I have heard several scare stories about it and am nervous about taking it. Can you tell me more about the pros and cons of this drug?*

A Most people taking antidepressant medication worry that it may cause their personality to change or their memory to suffer, and – worse – that they may become addicted to the drug. It is true that medication can cause unwanted side-effects or may not work as well as hoped. Fluoxetine (Prozac) is no exception, but its benefits tend to outweigh the disadvantages.

Prozac is one of a group of drugs known as serotonin re-uptake inhibitors (SSRIs), which increase the levels of the chemical serotonin (5HT) in the brain. It has proved to be a popular and effective antidepressant: it has fewer side-effects, interacts less with other drugs, and is less likely to cause death when taken in overdose than some older groups of antidepressant drugs. Prozac and other similar drugs are now widely used in the treatment of depression, and also for people with obsessive-compulsive disorders, bulimia, anxiety, phobias and severe PMS. The side-effects include anxiety, headaches, rashes, diarrhoea and difficulty in sleeping.

Prozac usually starts to work within a few days, but it could take a few weeks for the full effects of the medication to be felt. As with any other drug, if Prozac causes you to have any symptoms with which you are uncomfortable, or you feel worse after taking it, contact your doctor. When you are ready to stop the medication, discuss it with your doctor as it is better to tail it off than to stop abruptly.

It is important to remember that it is not an admission of defeat to take antidepressants. They may be an effective treatment for an otherwise debilitating bout of depression and if you find that they do not suit you, you can always stop or try another antidepressant, such as St John's wort, which is available without prescription. Antidepressants such as Prozac are not addictive and most people find it easy to come off them once their depressive illness has passed.

Q *Some time ago I fell into depression and was prescribed an antidepressant, amitriptyline. When I enquired about any side-effects I was told that there were no significant ones. A few days ago I was looking through a medical book, which listed the side-effects of various medicines, and was horrified to discover that there was a list half a page long; among them heart and blood problems, impotence, and so on. Should I stop using the medicine?*

A If you were to read about all the potential side-effects, cautions and interactions of any drug, you would never take so much as a paracetamol again and would flush any prescribed drug straight down the toilet, thinking the doctor was out to poison you. Of course, you do need to take note of the important warnings and major side-effects. A frank discussion with a pharmacist is always a good way of getting an informed perspective on any drug you are considering taking.

Amitriptyline (Lentizol) is not a trendy drug, unlike its more fashionable and younger rival, fluoxetine (Prozac). But it has been around for years, is effective and is safe so long as you do not overdose on it.

The drug's side-effects are largely predictable. It tends to make you tired, but that can be a good thing given that you usually take it at night and that sleep disturbance is often a feature of depression.

If you suffer from heart disease, glaucoma or prostate trouble, you probably should not be taking it and may want to discuss alternatives with your doctor. If amitriptyline is not helping your depression, you may want to try an antidepressant that works in a different way, such as the herbal remedy St John's wort, or discuss with your doctor whether drugs are actually what you need for the treatment of your depression.

Q *I have been suffering from mild depression and have nearly finished a course of antidepressants, which I was on for six weeks. I really do feel much better now, but am afraid that when the course has finished I may have a relapse and have to start again. How likely is this?*

A If you have suffered from depression, there is a chance that it will return. But with luck the circumstances that triggered your depression will have improved, and perhaps you have benefited from some counselling, or 'talking therapy', which will make a relapse less likely or severe if it does occur.

It does pay to come off antidepressants gradually if you have been on them for some time – although six weeks is not very long. Some people do just stop them suddenly, but this can lead to withdrawal effects, including dizziness, lethargy, pins and needles, and nausea. The longer you have been on your antidepressant, the more gradually you need to taper off – either by cutting pills in half, or taking the same dose but on alternate days. If you have been on Prozac (see above) for six months or more, you will be advised to reduce the dose by a quarter every four weeks.

If you did not consider counselling before, it may be a good idea to try it now.

Post-natal depression

Q *I became very depressed, weepy and panicky when my first baby was born 16 months ago. I am due to have another baby soon and am very worried that the same thing will happen. Is there anything I can do to guard against this?*

A It is totally normal for the initial euphoria of childbirth to give way to an emotional rollercoaster about three days after the birth. By day ten, you may be exhausted but should be happier. Post-natal depression (PND) is more rare and worse. It comes on about four to six weeks after the birth and can last for three to six months. It makes you feel low, anxious about being alone, unable to cope, uninterested in everything (including the baby), angry, guilty and troubled by ideas of harming the baby. Contrary to popular belief, PND is not caused by hormonal levels. It may be linked to previous bad labour, so talk through any unresolved fears with your midwife or obstetrician.

The more people you can rely on for psychological and practical support, the better. A support network including your partner, family, friends and local toddler groups, for example, will help to lessen the risk. Counselling to talk about underlying depression may be useful, and antidepressant drugs may be prescribed, even during pregnancy and breastfeeding, if you really need them. Having gone through PND once before, you are in a better position with this pregnancy: you know what to expect and will know to ask for help if you feel you are becoming depressed again. Useful resources are: the Meet A Mum Association★ Helpline (for details of self-help groups for mums with small kids), and the Association for Postnatal Illness,★ which enables women to share their experiences.

Premenstrual syndrome

Q *For up to two weeks every month, before my period, I feel emotionally unstable, irritable, often depressed, and behave quite unreasonably towards my husband and kids. I know this is due to premenstrual syndrome, and my doctor gave me an antidepressant (Prozac) for it, which did work, but I don't want to be on this until the menopause sets in. What else can I do?*

A Premenstrual syndrome (PMS) affects so many women that practically any remedy which is sold as a cure for PMS is bound to attract buyers. But both conventional medical and complementary therapies need to be taken with a pinch of salt, especially where extravagant claims are made for them.

True PMS is bad for up to two weeks before your period and gets better by the end of the period. If you are stressed or depressed all month, with a peak just before a period, you need to explore what is making you depressed and anxious, as it cannot all be due to your hormones. For true PMS, however, the following have been scientifically shown to be potentially beneficial:

- antidepressants, e.g. fluoxetine (Prozac), as you found
- anti-inflammatory painkillers, e.g. mefenamic acid (Ponstan)
- for tender breasts, the hormone-blocking drug danazol (Danol)
- for bloatedness and swelling, diuretics (water pills).

Treatments that may be beneficial are:

- vitamin B6
- evening primrose oil
- regular exercise
- oestrogen, e.g. as part of the contraceptive pill.

It is advisable to try the non-prescription, least harmful remedies or therapies first, i.e. regular exercise, vitamin B6 and evening primrose oil.

The National Association for Premenstrual Syndrome (NAPS)★ has a useful helpline.

Anxiety and stress

Q *My doctor has recently diagnosed me as suffering from anxiety attacks, and prescribed beta-blockers. I am a student nurse and feel that this is not correct. I do suffer from faintness and heart pounding, but this always occurs when I have really painful stomach cramps and diarrhoea. What do you think?*

A The physical symptoms of anxiety – palpitations, sweats and tremor – can also occur if you have an overactive thyroid (see Chapter 1) or if you take drugs containing adrenaline-like compounds or caffeine. Some over-the-counter cough and cold remedies may contain these products. You could try the following:

- cut out coffee, tea and cola, all of which contain caffeine
- do not take any over-the-counter medication at all for three weeks
- ask your GP for blood tests for anaemia and thyroid function
- ask yourself whether you are, indeed, anxious and whether you would like counselling or other psychological support to deal with it

- if anxiety *is* a problem, try to make a list of the triggers for your anxiety and tackle them one by one – for example, seeing your tutor about work pressure, if that is a contributing cause
- resort to the beta-blockers only if the physical symptoms of anxiety are intense and interfering with your daily life. If they make you dizzy, however, you may wish to refrain from them altogether.

Q *I work as an infant teacher and have felt off-colour for most of this term. It is a small school and providing cover for sick teachers is a nightmare. We are under enormous pressure to turn up for work even when ill. I wonder whether I should push myself to go in even when, as last week, I had raging tonsillitis, or look after myself and take a few days off, as my GP recommends. Will my health suffer in the long term if I keep pushing myself?*

A The results of a recent study in Sweden show that people who go to work when ill do not recuperate properly and end up taking more sick leave and feeling unwell for longer periods. The study of 3,801 people found that teachers, nurses, childminders and carers have the highest rates of turning up to work when sick. These are also the groups that have the poorest long-term health, with high rates of mild depression, fatigue and back pain. Interestingly, the study also showed that age and education are not indicators of who shows up for work and who does not.

Phobias and social problems

Q *I have developed a very severe phobia about heights, to the extent that I can no longer use an escalator and get panic-stricken if I go in one of those glass lifts where you can see down. This fear is beginning to seriously damage my ability to live a normal life. Can you explain why it might be happening and what I can do about it?*

A It is estimated that nearly one in ten people has an extreme fear (or phobia) of something – heights, lifts, spiders, etc. Having a phobia means that while you are fine most of the time, you experience intense anxiety if you come into contact with the object or situation that triggers your fear. This makes you go to enormous lengths to avoid exposure and this avoidance can become very debilitating.

You may know rationally that you are not going to fall off a high place, lifts will not trap you forever and spiders cannot hurt you, but that does not stop it being a very frightening thing for you.

Phobias usually arise out of the blue and often there is no one traumatic event to explain it. It may seem silly or embarrassing to explain your phobia even to close family or friends, and some people battle on with phobias without sharing their anxiety with anyone. That is a shame, because you can do quite a lot to help yourself – say, talking about your fear to someone you can trust, joining a self-help group, learning a relaxation technique such as yoga, or having specific counselling. Cognitive behavioural therapy is probably the most effective 'talking therapy' (see start of this chapter for details) for phobias. Medication includes tranquillisers in the very short term for acute panic attacks, but they are addictive and therefore not suitable in the longer term. Beta-blockers can block the physical signs of anxiety (e.g. palpitations) and antidepressants can be useful especially if the phobia has contributed to more generalised depression.

Further advice is available from the National Phobic Society.★

Q *I have very low self-esteem and constantly think people are talking about me behind my back. I hear them call me nasty names and when I accuse them of doing it they deny it. I have a tendency to talk to myself and am afraid to go out and mix with people. All of this means that I have not been able to hold a job down for any length of time. I do not want to take medication for my problem. Is there anything else I can do to help myself?*

A It is understandable that you do not want to take medication but that is no reason not to seek expert and sympathetic advice, initially from your GP. Your low self-esteem is clearly upsetting you and affecting your lifestyle and ability to make and keep friends. It is possible for you to get help and confidence with some treatment that does not involve drugs.

Your first step should be to explore with your GP the nature and causes of your condition. You may find that your problem is a result of:

• depression or anxiety

- a mild communication disorder such as Asperger's syndrome which makes it hard for you to interact with people
- a particular personality type which makes you suspicious of others and awkward in social situations
- a tendency to schizophrenia.

Of course, it may turn out that you have none of these and may just be a shy person whose confidence needs boosting.

You will be able to choose from a range of options such as seeing a psychiatrist, a counsellor one to one, attending a group for people with similar problems, trying medication if you wish, or being followed up closely by your doctor.

Q *I have always been shy, but I am becoming increasingly self-conscious and worried about going out or meeting new people. I try to avoid situations in which I might be the centre of attention and have even started making excuses rather than going out with friends, in case we meet new people and I am forced to make conversation with them. I become very anxious if I know I am likely to have to talk in a group at work – for instance, at team meetings. I blush very readily and then become embarrassed that I am deep red. My reluctance to speak up is hampering my prospects at work. What is wrong with me?*

A Most of us feel shy in some circumstances and blush if very embarrassed. Shyness becomes a problem only when – as in your case – it is causing you distress and possibly stopping you from enjoying life to the full and achieving your potential in the workplace and socially. It is then called a social phobia. It is estimated that three in a hundred women and one in a hundred men experience this type of social phobia.

Sometimes blushing and shyness may be accompanied by physical signs of anxiety, such as sweating and palpitations. In extreme cases, people may also have panic attacks and feel faint or breathless, and have a tingling sensation in their fingers.

Most intensely shy people arrange their lives so as not to be in stressful situations. If you cannot do this without feeling that your life is becoming unduly restricted, or if you are depressed by your phobia, you can take measures to help yourself. You could, for example, go on an assertiveness-training course, which is arranged by some local authorities, psychological medicine departments in large hospitals and adult education centres. Your GP, local library, nearest adult education centre or MIND* can give you information on such courses. Counselling, either one-to-one or in a group, can help a great deal. In terms of medication, beta-blockers could be prescribed to relieve the physical effects of anxiety-like palpitations. Tranquillisers (e.g. diazepam – Valium) should be avoided if possible because they are potentially addictive and can impair short-term memory. A group of antidepressants known as monoamine oxidase inhibitors (MAOIs) can be useful. In the past they interacted with many other drugs and some foods and so were not suitable for everyone. Newer types of MAOIs have fewer limitations on their use. Another group of antidepressants which has been found to be helpful in treating social phobias includes fluoxetine (Prozac) – see page 48.

Surviving abuse

Q *I was sexually abused as a child. The perpetrator was an older male relative, and although I am certain that my mother suspected what was going on, she never confronted him or protected me. I have suppressed my awful memories, and although I might appear to cope well with daily life, the price for this semblance of normality has been high. I have two wonderful children and a loving partner, but I am constantly testing his love and am riddled with insecurities. My self-esteem is terrible and I suffer dreadful anxieties on behalf of my children. I am worried that I will wreck my marriage and alienate my children as they get older unless I can sort myself out. Can you help?*

A You have emerged from a very dark shadow and built a loving home for your husband and children which is totally different from the one in which you grew up. You should congratulate yourself for having overcome the odds and got this far, and use the confidence you gain from acknowledging this to seek expert help in dealing with the deep trauma that still haunts you. Your GP should be able to recommend an experienced therapist, or you could contact a support organisation such as Family Matters.*

You are not alone, as you know. It is now recognised that abuse is very widespread, with as many as one in four girls and one in six boys being sexually abused, in some way, before they reach the age of 18.

Sexual abuse in childhood causes lasting damage, but people like yourself can recover and become whole again. Abuse at a young age robs people of their innocence, damages their ability to trust others and often leads to low self-esteem and an inability to form meaningful sexual relationships later in life. Moreover, the early experience of having their trust shattered may mean that they doubt their ability to make sound decisions or judgements about others. Panic attacks, anxiety, feelings of isolation and despair are all common among survivors of abuse.

Talking therapies (see page 44) can help you to explore some of the residual self-doubts that are your legacy from the years of abuse. Many abusers tell their impressionable victims that there is no harm in what they are doing and that the child must never tell anyone. They may even suggest that the child had it coming to him ore her or in some way invited the abuse. As an adult, you may recognise that these sentiments are wrong, manipulative and designed to shield the abuser. But they may have left a lasting impression that is hard to shrug off, and therapy can aid you to do this.

Therapy will also allow you to express the hurt, anger, sense of betrayal and mourning for lost childhood that you undoubtedly feel. You will be able to recognise how the abuse has left you vulnerable emotionally and how you can unpick the hurt and rebuild your own personality. This is a voyage of recovery, not an overnight redemption and the path can be long and painful. Learning to trust those you love most, and to rely on friends, colleagues and your therapist may all take time. You may find that key events in your own adult life present new challenges: dealing with the death of your abuser, confronting family members, such as your mother, who may have shielded your abuse and so on may all prove formative but very challenging.

With the passage of time, and a lot of work on your part, you can recover. In the process you will learn a lot about yourself, become empowered and perhaps emerge a better parent, lover and friend to others.

Eating disorders

Q *When I met my girlfriend 18 months ago I was amazed by how healthy her attitude to food was. More than any girl I'd ever met she ate what she wanted. She had suffered from anorexia and bulimia in her adolescence and dealt with it then. But now she has become very thin again, and she realises that this is a recurrence of the anorexia (she assures me she is not making herself sick). We have talked about it a lot, and I know she vacillates between tolerance of her condition and despair at its re-emergence. I want to help but have no idea how to. Can you advise me?*

A She is lucky to have your love and concern. You are forcing her to confront a problem that clearly needs addressing urgently. Your role is to stand by and support her but not to take on the entire burden of getting her appropriate treatment. She needs to be referred to a unit specialising in eating disorders, which will be able to offer expert help. Her GP should know about local resources and can refer her to an NHS unit. Private care is available, but is rarely covered by health insurance and can be extremely costly for the sort of long-term follow-up she will need.

The following guidance may be helpful.

- The first step is for the sufferer to identify and recognise his or her problem.
- Binge eaters (see opposite) often find self-help books useful. Seeing a GP or practice-based nurse, dietician or counsellor once a fortnight for around three months can help to provide support and encouragement. Up to 50 per cent of binge eaters will recover this way; others may respond better to a group or an eating disorders specialist.
- Those with bulimia (see opposite) are best helped by cognitive behavioural therapy (CBT). This involves a step-by-step recovery programme, which can be undertaken using a book or, preferably, with the assistance of a trained counsellor. Most programmes take 12 weeks to complete.
- People suffering from anorexia (see opposite) usually need specialist help and more intensive therapy. The sufferer should certainly be referred to a specialist if his or her BMI (see page 16) is under 17.5, as very serious medical problems, such as dehydration and metabolic abnormalities in the short term, and osteoporosis in the long term, need addressing.

Eating disorders

Types of eating disorders:

- **binge eating** refers to eating more food in a given period of time than most people would, resulting in a feeling of loss of control. Binge eaters do not usually use weight-controlling measures such as vomiting
- **anorexia nervosa** is an over-concern with shape and weight and an intense fear of becoming fat. Strict dieting, excessive exercise and sometimes vomiting are used to keep weight abnormally low. Periods may stop for at least three months at a time
- **bulimia nervosa** also involves over-concern with shape and weight, frequent binges and extreme measures to prevent weight gain, such as vomiting, laxatives, fasting and diuretics (water pills). Weight is usually in the normal range.

The following criteria can be used to identify whether someone has an eating disorder:

- abnormal methods of weight control: always dieting, vomiting after eating, using laxatives and diuretics when not medically necessary, and extreme exercise
- obsessive attitude to shape and weight: deeply unhappy with weight and shape, such that nothing is more important
- extreme eating habits: episodes of loss of control of eating; binge eating
- weight: excessively low body mass index (BMI – see page 16), i.e. under 17.5.

- People with co-existing problems such as depression, alcoholism, drug abuse and medical conditions such as diabetes should receive expert attention urgently. Any eating disorder that has persisted for over six months, despite attempts to overcome it with self-help techniques, requires specialist advice sooner rather than later.

Support and advice is available from the Eating Disorders Association.*

Mental illness

Schizophrenia

Q *I have a close friend who has been behaving strangely in the past few weeks. She has become unconcerned about her appearance, frequently going to work looking dishevelled, and says she hears voices telling her what to do. Her parents have suggested that she probably has schizophrenia, and have arranged for her to see a doctor. In the meantime, I would like to know more about the condition. What are its main characteristics and how can we help her should schizophrenia be diagnosed?*

A Schizophrenia is a mental illness that can be helped but not cured. It affects one in a hundred people and usually becomes apparent when a person leaves school and starts to be more independent. The younger a person is when diagnosed with schizophrenia, the more likely he or she is to have problems coping with everyday life. It is a distressing illness for the individual and family, friends and colleagues. A person suffering from the condition can find it difficult to study, work, form permanent relationships and communicate with others. He or she may have periods of relatively good mental health and intermittent relapses which may be triggered by stress or come on out of the blue.

The essential problem is that a person with schizophrenia suffers a dissociation from reality as the rest of the world would perceive it. This can lead to a disturbed and troubled state of mind, and behaviour and speech that is hard for most people to understand or follow.

A person with schizophrenia may feel as though his or her mind and body have been taken over by some outside, alien force which is controlling him or her and putting thoughts into his or her mind. This can be very frightening and confusing. He or she may hear voices – like your friend – or see, smell or feel something that is not actually there. The person may also have delusions or false ideas which he or she will not relinquish even in the face of what others would recognise as firm evidence to the contrary. He or she may believe that the whole world is conspiring against him or her and be very upset. Arguing with such a person and trying to convince him or her that the ideas are false or that there are no voices will not help, as his or her idea of reality is different from yours when he or she is unwell.

The distorted sense of reality also accounts for the way that some people suffering from schizophrenia retreat from mainstream life. A person with the condition may – again, like your friend – become increasingly unkempt, unwashed, untidy and lethargic. He or she may not be motivated enough to make any social contacts and may become increasingly reclusive. People around him or her may find that his or her conversation is bizarre and that it is impossible to follow his or her train of thought; moreover, he or she may talk more to the voices than to members of his or her own family as the voices may seem more real to him or her.

The most effective way of helping your friend is to support and love her, and to encourage her to take her medication and get expert help when she is distressed or clearly not coping. Do not remonstrate with her and try to get her to change the way she is behaving and living. Also, remember that the majority of people with schizophrenia are not dangerous. However, they do have an increased danger of self-harm, and to a lesser extent of harming others.

As mentioned earlier, there is no cure for schizophrenia, but the outlook for those with the condition can be positive. After a first bout of schizophrenia, one-quarter of people make a good recovery within five years. Most (two-thirds) will tend to have ups and downs and will not be able to function well in mainstream life without special support. Less than 10 per cent will not recover and will be incapacitated by their condition.

For further advice and support contact the National Schizophrenia Fellowship★ or MIND.★

Q *My brother has just been diagnosed as schizophrenic. This is very upsetting for our family – we don't really know what to think and can't help wondering if we are to blame in any way. What causes schizophrenia? And what is the treatment?*

A No one knows for certain what causes schizophrenia although countless theories have been advanced over the years. Often when someone is diagnosed as having schizophrenia, no one else in his or her family is known to have the condition. But in about half of all cases, there is thought to be an inherited component, though scientists have not yet identified the gene that is responsible for schizophrenia. Developmental theories suggest that schizophrenia occurs when the brain does not develop properly either because of infections while in the womb or damage while being born.

A first attack of schizophrenia or relapses may be triggered by traumatic events such as a bereavement. Addictive drugs such as LSD, amphetamines and alcohol do not cause schizophrenia but, like stress, may trigger or exacerbate the condition.

Treatment of the first episode often takes place under the care of a psychiatrist in hospital. Admission is usually necessary for a formal assessment and treatment plan to be worked out with the individual and his or her family. Drugs (antipsychotics) are used to alleviate symptoms though they will not cure the condition. Social workers, psychiatric nurses, psychiatrists, occupational therapists and other health professionals ideally work as a team to discuss the patient's housing, benefits, work, day-time activities and rehabilitation. Counselling helps and usually focuses on understanding and modifying behaviour. The ongoing support and involvement of family and close friends is important, though carers need a respite from time to time as the ongoing responsibility may be very wearing.

People with schizophrenia may not have insight into their condition and may refuse treatment when they need it most. The Mental Health Act in England and Wales and similar legislation in the rest of Britain allows compulsory admission to hospital if the person is a danger to him- or herself or others or urgently needs treatment.

Manic depression

Q *My father, whom I never knew, apparently suffered from manic depression. I am very concerned that I may have inherited a tendency to it. Is it hereditary? What are the signs?*

A Psychiatric terms are often used very loosely in families, so it may be useful for you to find out whether your father truly had manic depression or just an up-and-down temperament. If he had manic depression, he may have spent time in hospital, been under the care of a psychiatrist and taken medication called lithium throughout his life. Moreover, although manic depression can run in families, you are by no means certain to have inherited it even if your father was affected.

The underlying problem in manic depression seems to be that parts of the brain controlling mood do not work properly. No one gene has yet been found to be the cause of this, nor one chemical in the brain implicated. Episodes of manic depression may be triggered by stressful events including physical illness or being made redundant, but they probably do not cause the problem.

About one in a hundred people suffers from manic depression at some point in their lives. It affects men as often as women. The condition causes wild mood swings and extremes of behaviour which can be damaging both to the individual and others.

In a depressed, or down, phase, a person with manic depression suffers from a lack of enjoyment in anything, feelings of uselessness and despair, inability to concentrate and make decisions, disturbed sleep and appetite, and loss of libido. He or she may even feel suicidal and is at risk of suicide when very down.

In a manic, or up, phase, he or she may feel unusually full of energy and excitement, be unable to sleep, be bubbling with ideas and feel particularly generous and capable of doing anything. He or she may also hear voices but they are usually less disturbing than the voices that a schizophrenic may be plagued by. The problem with the manic phase is that although some surges of energy and excitement may be creative and productive, mania loosens a person's grip on reality. To the outsider, someone in the manic phase may seem very attractive but may rapidly become a liability. Behaviour can become bizarre and unacceptable to most people and words may come out under such pressure as to be unintelligible. The person may act in a sexually promiscuous way, spend money recklessly and be so 'over the top' that he or she is no longer employable. Relationships may be wrecked during the manic phase and may be severely tested in the depressed phase. There may be long periods of time in between when mood swings level out and behaviour is less extreme.

Depression is helped by counselling and antidepressants. Most manic depressives derive benefit from lithium, a drug that levels out mood swings. Weight gain is the most common side-effect of taking lithium and regular blood tests are needed to make sure the dose is correct. Psychiatrists, community psychiatric nurses, social workers, GPs and occupational therapists may all help with managing the condition. Close friends and family who know how to spot the signs of drastic mood swings, and can contact the professional services if the individual will not or cannot, are invaluable and need to be involved in the care of the manic-depressive person.

Contact the Manic Depression Fellowship★ or MIND★ for further advice.

Syndromes

Obsessive-compulsive disorder

Q *My 12-year-old son has been exhibiting increasingly neurotic behaviour over the past few months. He has become obsessed with following strict rituals in his everyday life and gets very distressed when other members of the family do not join in. I have heard of something called obsessive-compulsive disorder. Could this be what is the matter with him? If so, how can he be helped?*

A Lots of children have habits and ritual behaviour that become emphasised when they are stressed or under pressure, e.g. twitching, screwing up eyes, biting nails, pulling out eyelashes, washing hands repeatedly, and so on. It is worthwhile discussing with your son whether something is bothering him at school: is he being bullied, or finding the academic pressure too much? Is there tension at home between you and your partner or conflict with an older sibling that may be upsetting him? If you can identify a trigger, it would be better to deal with that rather than focusing on his behaviour.

Obsessions are ideas and recurring thoughts that keep coming into your mind even though you try to push them out. The thoughts may be persistent, upsetting or even frightening and you may even know that they do not make sense.

Compulsions are actions that you feel you have to do even though you do not want to. Many of us, including children, have mild compulsions or rituals which can be comforting in their familiarity – having a particular way of arranging ornaments, certificates, or books, for instance. A five-year old who lines up her teddies in a certain order every night does not have a problem. But a 12-year-old who cannot go to school in the morning because he has to wash his hands 20 times in a particular and very time-consuming way does.

A person whose compulsions get in the way of his or her functioning normally or who becomes very disturbed or anxious when he or she cannot give in to the compulsion is said to be suffering from obsessive-compulsive disorder (OCD).

No one knows for sure what causes OCD. One theory is that an imbalance of the chemical serotonin in the brain may be responsible for it. It is possible that OCD is an inherited tendency because it can run in families. OCD can affect people of all ages though it is often not diagnosed until adult life. Probably one in a hundred teenagers is affected. It seems that early diagnosis and treatment can be helpful so it is best not to wait until adult patterns of behaviour set in.

If you think your son may have OCD, go and discuss it with your GP. You may want to request referral to a child and adolescent psychiatrist for an expert assessment. Other underlying problems such as depression can also be picked up and treated. You will want to discuss the situation with your son's teachers and see what help the school can offer.

The two most effective treatments for OCD are cognitive behavioural therapy (see above) and anti-depressant medication to boost serotonin levels (e.g. fluoxetine or Prozac and clomipramine or Anafranil). The combination of the two can be extremely effective.

For further advice, contact MIND.*

Asperger's syndrome

Q *For many years we have been concerned that there is something wrong with our ten-year-old child, as he cannot interact with his classmates normally and has always been a loner. Now he has been diagnosed as having Asperger's syndrome. What does this mean and how can we help him?*

A Finding out that your son has a specific condition which explains some aspects of his behaviour may have come as something of a relief to you. At least now you can seek and get focused help.

Asperger's syndrome (or disorder) affects a person's social skills and interaction with others. It is sometimes thought of as being on the same spectrum as autism though it tends to cause less severe problems than autism. No one really knows what causes Asperger's although it may run in families to a certain extent. It is unlikely that any one gene causes the syndrome.

A child with *autism* usually starts speaking only after the age of two and may have severe language delay. He or she may suffer from impaired intelligence and his or her behaviour may be markedly abnormal and difficult to deal with.

On the other hand, a child with *Asperger's* usually starts to talk by two, has normal intelligence and shows behavioural patterns that are unusual but less disruptive than a child with autism.

This may explain why it can be hard to diagnose Asperger's: the problems may be subtle and not become manifest until nursery or school age. People with Asperger's are often called 'loners', as you say your son is. You may find that he is very self-sufficient, content to busy himself in apparently pointless and repetitive activities such as lining up books in order of height over and over again. He may not demand much attention from you and indeed may become upset and frustrated if his solitude is disturbed.

Your son will be under the overall care of a team led by a child psychiatrist, preferably one with some expertise of Asperger's. They will monitor his progress, coordinate resources such as social services, and work with you and your family to develop programmes to help him. Medication is not usually necessary but can be used if other problems crop up (e.g. if your son becomes depressed, agitated or anxious). Apart from seeking professional help, you can help in other ways, too. Ask his teacher at school what he is like in class: is he happy, or shy, or is he bullied? Would having a classroom assistant working alongside him help him?

Your son is not a label. He is as unique as every other child. He will probably encounter some problems in his interactions with peers, and may find it harder than some kids to make friends and sustain long-term relationships in the future. But the help that he will get now will encourage him to read social situations better and should make it easier for him to overcome any natural barriers he has so that he can function fully and independently as an adult.

For more information, contact the National Autistic Society★ or the Dyscovery Centre.★

Autism

Q *I'm desperately worried about my three-year-old son. He is a very solitary little boy who prefers his own company, even to mine. His speech is reasonable but he doesn't speak much and seems to live in a world of his own. He started nursery recently which I was hoping would make him more sociable but the nursery teachers say he plays on his own and gets very upset if interrupted.*

With all this talk about the safety of the MMR [measles, mumps, rubella] vaccine (which he had), I'm concerned that he may be autistic. My husband doesn't think there's anything to worry about and says he's just a shy little boy who needs time to develop. How can I find out if there's anything wrong?

A The first thing you should realise before you seek expert help on whether your son has autism is that the supposed link between the MMR immunisation and autism does not appear to be founded on good scientific evidence, although many parents and some health professionals are clearly concerned about it. A study reported in September 2001 by researchers at St George's Hospital and the Institute of Child Health (both in London) drew reassuring conclusions about the safety of the vaccine, and said that no evidence was found to support the claim that giving the vaccines singly is safer and more effective (see also Chapter 11).

If this does not reassure you, and you do not think your husband is right that your son is merely shy, it is best you get professional advice to put an end to your uncertainty.

Start by contacting the National Autistic Society (NAS)★, and ask for its checklist for autism in toddlers; another version that you can request is one used by health professionals. These checklists provide a useful indicator as to whether you have grounds for concern.

The next step is to speak to your health visitor and GP and ask for referral to a community paediatrician for an assessment. Early diagnosis opens the door to professional support and educational assistance and helps your child to progress, so do not be fobbed off until you are satisfied that your son has had an expert assessment.

Autism affects a person's communication with others, thereby impeding social interactions. It often manifests itself in repetitive behaviour that may limit his or her potential. The condition affects up to four times as many boys as girls. An autistic child or adult is unable to respond fully to others. He or she may not show any interest even if a companion suddenly bursts into tears, because he or she cannot understand social cues that most of us would pick up. The autistic person may therefore come across as grossly insensitive, uncaring or badly behaved, but one should not interpret his or her behaviour as such. To an autistic person it can seem as if everyone is speaking a totally foreign language: he or she may understand the individual words but can make no sense of the situation. All of this makes it hard to bond with an autistic child. Loving parents may become frustrated and sad that their love appears to be unwelcome to the child and is not returned. Their attempts to play with their child are rebuffed or ignored. The routines and rituals that autistic children crave can be very disruptive for the rest of the family. The autistic child may become very agitated when his or her routine is disturbed so that the whole family ends up sacrificing flexibility and spontaneity for a quieter life. Siblings can often adapt better to the autistic child than adults can but problems can crop up as the siblings move into adolescence. Autistic children may often seem unhappy in themselves and may harm themselves, develop phobias and become very anxious. Mainstream schooling with support may be possible but about three-quarters of children with autism have learning difficulties. Indeed, despite a commonly held view, few autistic children have the remarkable skills of so-called *idiots savants*, such as the one portrayed by Dustin Hoffman in the film *Rain Man*.

Autistic children grow into autistic adults with difficulties forming relationships, finding jobs and communicating with others. But recognition of the problems and expert skills training can yield wonderful results, so a diagnosis of autism need not be a wholly negative blow.

Tourette's syndrome

Q *My 13-year-old son is a serious worry to me. He makes little jerky movements with his head which he seems to be able to stop if we tell him to, but which recur in a flurry after a few minutes. He has some learning difficulties for which he is helped at school, but his attention span is very limited. He gets on OK socially although I think he is a bit of a loner. Our GP says he seems to be a normal adolescent, but once she saw the head movements said she would refer him to a specialist to see if he has something called Tourette's syndrome. We are still waiting for an appointment and I am very concerned to find out more about this syndrome and whether my son might have it. What is it?*

A The first thing to say is that your son may just have developed a rather persistent habit. If no one else in your family is known to have had similar movements, Tourette's is unlikely as it is usually an inherited condition.

Tourette's syndrome (TS) is diagnosed on the basis of symptoms: no specific tests are available for it yet. Those who have it tend suddenly to shout out rude and inappropriate words (a habit not uncommon to many 'normal' teenagers) accompanied by abnormal jerky movements known as tics. Learning difficulties are common too.

Nobody knows what causes TS but it is thought to be due in part to the brain's inability to control the chemical responsible for movement, known as dopamine. One theory is that in genetically susceptible individuals, a bacterial infection such as streptococcus, which is responsible for tonsillitis and ear infections, may trigger off a reaction by the body's immune system that results in damage.

TS is usually fairly mild and there is no one cure. It can be useful to have the diagnosis made so that your son can explain to others that he is not mad or bad but has a condition that makes him twitch and swear uncontrollably.

He will benefit from behavioural therapy to modify his swearing and behaviour and may need more long-term therapy to help boost his self-confidence. People who have TS can sometimes be taught to override their tics or redirect them into some other less obtrusive movement. A range of medications can be tried but no single drug is guaranteed to work.

People with TS find that the tics are often worst in their early teens and then improve. About a third of people with TS lose their tics altogether in adult life though they cannot be certain they will not return later. Some sufferers find their tics much better in adulthood, while others continue to experience troublesome symptoms throughout life.

For more information, contact the Tourette's Syndrome Association.★

Memory loss and dementia

Q *I had a fairly severe bout of glandular fever six years ago at the age of 17. During my illness I noticed that my short-term memory was virtually non-existent. I couldn't for the life of me remember what I had said to people during conversations from the previous day. I still have a terrible short-term memory and I can't remember whether I have completed tasks, told someone something or even brushed my teeth in the morning! I read somewhere that this can be a side-effect of glandular fever. Is this true and should I still be affected now?*

A Short-term memory is not known to be affected by glandular fever. In severe cases, there can be some inflammation of the brain (encephalitis), which causes confusion at the time of the illness, but normally people recover fully without any memory impairment. It may be that your concentration has lapsed since you have been ill and that you are finding it hard to focus on memorising things. Sometimes the more you worry about memory, the harder it is to remember new information. You can test your short-term memory against friends or relatives by playing memory games (such as putting a certain number of items on a tray, removing it from sight and then writing down as many items as you can remember). Try to retrain your memory by setting yourself small manageable tasks, such as learning a short poem by heart. You will probably find that the less you think about it, the better your memory will be.

Q *There is a long history of multi-infarct dementia in my family. The thought that I could get it terrifies me. What measures can I take to avoid it?*

A Multi-infarct dementia (MID), which is caused by a series of mini-strokes restricting the blood supply to the brain, is not known to be inherited in any predictable way. There is also a fair bit you can do to try to minimise your own risk of developing MID or related diseases, such as heart attacks and strokes (see Chapter 1). The single most important factor is not to smoke. Get your blood pressure, cholesterol and blood sugar levels checked by your GP and make sure they are all kept within normal range, if necessary by taking medication. Ask the GP to check your pulse rate and listen to your heart, because irregular heartbeats can throw off small blood clots (emboli), which can contribute to MID.

Whether a daily aspirin will help prevent dementia is debatable. On balance, the risk of the aspirin causing stomach ulcers and bleeding may outweigh any potential benefits.

Q *I am 65 and my memory is awful. I am desperately worried that I'm getting Alzheimer's, as my mother did in her eighties, and every time I can't find a word I get in a terrible state. How do I know when it is dementia? It is making me very low and panicky.*

A Dementia (progressive memory loss) is uncommon in people of 65, although it affects one in five people over the age of 80. It is hardly ever inherited, so there is no particular reason for you to go the same way as your mother.

Poor memory can also be a sign of being a bit depressed, although mild depression may be missed more often in older than younger people, because it is assumed that forgetfulness is an inevitable part of old age, which it is not! People of all ages have memory lapses, but our awareness of them and concern about them grows as we get older.

Because Alzheimer's, which accounts for half of all cases of dementia, causes gradual memory loss and disorientation, the sufferer is usually the last to be aware of his or her symptoms. Your GP will be able to ask you a series of questions to test your memory, carry out some simple urine and blood tests, and refer you to a specialist if dementia is suspected. If you are depressed, you can discuss treatment options.

Stammering

Q *I am now a successful businessman in my thirties but have been plagued all my life by a tendency to stammer when I'm under pressure. I recently had some feedback from work colleagues that my stammer counts against me when I am presenting to clients. I was very upset by this as I thought I was accepted for who and what I am and that my stammer is just part of me. I've never had any particular help except some brief speech therapy when I was young, which my mother says did help at the time. Why do I stammer and is there anything I can do about it?*

A We are all less fluent in our speech at some times than others. Most people who stammer do not do so all the time, and few people stammer in exactly the same way. Stress, tiredness and certain methods of communication, such as the phone, may trigger stammering, while at other times you are more fluent. Speech and language therapists can help a great deal if you feel you have a problem. It is quite possible that if it does not bother you, it is not bothering your clients, and that for some reason your colleagues are being malicious.

No single answer can be given as to why some people stammer, because there is no single type of stammer, nor any one type of person who stammers. The most likely answer is that stammering is caused by a combination of factors rather than just one issue.

You may believe that if you can find out why you stammer, you will find a cure. We know that more men than women stammer, that there is a 20 per cent greater chance of your stammering if a close relative has a speech problem, that stammerers often had some difficulty with learning the words or sounds of speech in early childhood, and that emotional stress on a child can be an issue.

While considering these factors you may realise that, whatever might have caused your stammer, identifying the reason is really of little help because you will have gone through substantial changes since those early childhood days.

Expert advice is available from the British Stammering Association.*

Shaking hands

Q *My hands shake uncontrollably sometimes, though at other times they are fine. I am in good general health but this worries me. I am scared that it might be a sign of Parkinson's disease. What else could it be?*

A The chances are that your hands shake when you are anxious. The commonest type of shaking hands (tremor) is due to anxiety, alcohol, drugs or an overactive thyroid (see Chapter 1). In addition to tremor, symptoms of anxiety include palpitations and sweats. You may want to discuss your alcohol intake and any medication with your GP, to see whether these could be contributing to the tremor. A blood test can tell you whether your thyroid is overactive.

An inherited cause of tremor is known as 'benign essential tremor'. Involuntary movements of both arms and head are usual, and improve when you drink alcohol. Although the condition is inherited, it can start at any age. The drug propranolol (Inderal) helps in at least a third of cases. Rarer causes of tremors that become more exaggerated when you try to reach out for something can be due to damage to the part of the brain known as the cerebellum, in conditions such as multiple sclerosis (see Chapter 1).

Shaking hands that are worse when you are not doing anything can be a sign of early Parkinson's disease (see box opposite). This tends to come on over the age of about 65, and affects many aspects of movement, including gait. One of the first signs is sometimes that your handwriting gets progressively smaller when you write a letter. Drug treatment and physiotherapy may help to control the symptoms.

Parkinson's disease

Parkinson's disease is a progressive neurological condition characterised by shaking (tremor), stiffness (rigidity) and slowness of movement. People who suffer from Parkinsonism find that their movements become slow, their hands shake especially when resting, their handwriting gets smaller, they take short, shuffling steps which makes it look like they are about to fall forward, and their facial expressions become fixed and expressionless. Dribbling may be a problem too. Symptoms can vary from hour to hour and day to day.

The condition is caused by a lack of dopamine, the chemical in the brain responsible for movement. Parkinson's disease results from the degeneration of the nerves in the brain that produce dopamine. Symptoms usually start between the ages of 60 and 70, and one in 200 people over the age of 65 is affected. Some drugs used for nausea and in the treatment of schizophrenia can cause similar symptoms. Stopping the drugs or counteracting them with others (e.g. procyclidine or Kemadrin) can reverse the Parkinsonism.

A neurologist confirms the diagnosis and together with the GP can advise about treatment. Drug treatment aims to replace the falling dopamine levels. The dosage has to be tailored to the individual and may need frequent readjustment. The aim is to find the lowest dose of drug needed to control symptoms and avoid side-effects. Drugs (such as Madopar and Sinemet) combine the active ingredient, L-dopa (a form of dopamine), with a chemical that prevents side-effects to parts of the body outside the brain.

Depression is a common problem and should also be treated with counselling and/or anti-depressants. Occupational therapists can help fit aids in the home, social services can provide financial benefits and admission into day centres, and physiotherapists can improve mobility and balance.

Restless legs

Q *When I have to keep still for any length of time I get a deep feeling in my leg muscles, which is not exactly painful but is very unpleasant, and causes a violent urge to move my legs around. It is very embarrassing when I am out somewhere, like the cinema or a restaurant, as it is quite uncontrollable. I tried quinine, which my doctor said was good for cramps, but it didn't work and I wouldn't really describe the feeling as cramps. What on earth is it? Is there anything I can do about it?*

A Your problem is graced by its own name – Ekbom's syndrome, otherwise known as restless legs syndrome (RLS). No one knows what causes it, although some defect in part of the brain responsible for movement, the basal ganglia, has been suggested. Many drugs and complementary therapies have been tried, most of which do not work. The drug carbamazepine (Tegretol), which is used in some forms of epilepsy and other neurological conditions, may be worth trying. The condition is not dangerous and does not predispose you to any more serious problems – it is just a nuisance. There is in fact a Restless Legs Syndrome Foundation,★ which can offer help and provide contact with other sufferers via its web site.

Chapter 3

Sexual matters

No couple can sustain a long relationship without the odd hiccup in their sex life, and many external factors may affect a person's sex drive and performance. Sex is not a prerequisite of a successful relationship (couples may lovingly and mutually agree to stop having intercourse) and neither is it a reliable indicator of a healthy relationship (it might be satisfying for one partner but not the other, or could be a weapon within an abusive or destructive relationship). Whatever the context, sexual problems will arise when reality does not match the expectations of one or both partners.

Most sexual problems have more than one cause. Physical, psychological and social factors often interact to create a problem. Examples of physical causes are tiredness, side-effects of medication, alcohol, heart disease and diabetes. Psychological causes may include depression, anxiety, previous rape or abuse, expectation of sexual failure or uncertainty about sexual orientation. The lack of privacy in a small house with several children is an example of a social cause.

The most common sexual problems for men are impotence (an inability to get an erection) and premature ejaculation ('coming' too quickly). For women, the most common problems are vaginismus (muscles spasm making the vagina too tight for intercourse) and an inability to reach orgasm. For both men and women, low sex drive, pain during intercourse, unresolved feelings or previous negative experiences can get in the way of a satisfying sexual relationship.

This chapter offers advice and guidance about all these predicaments. It also covers sexually transmitted diseases, including HIV, and discusses safe sex practices. It includes a look at transsexualism, and suggests how to get help in dealing with deviant sexual behaviour. Owing to the limitations of space, this chapter focuses largely on heterosexual sex, but it does give some advice about coming to terms with homosexual orientation.

Details of support organisations are provided at the back of the book. Adolescents and young adults may find the advice and counselling available from the Brook Advisory Centres★ particularly useful.

Treatment and help

Even the most fleeting of sexual encounters does not happen in a vacuum. Sex happens within a relationship, however transient, and in addressing a sexual problem we must consider how it affects and is affected by that relationship. This means appreciating all the contributing factors and not jumping to conclusions. Lack of sex drive does not necessarily mean he is having an affair, tight vaginal muscles does not always mean she does not want to have sex with you, impotence does not signify failure, and premature ejaculation is not a measure of immaturity or selfishness. Rushing out to get Viagra may buy you an erection, but is not a substitute for exploring with your partner the reasons why you are not getting an erection when you want one.

Many of us attribute sexual problems to hormonal imbalance, such as lack of testosterone in men or menopausal changes in women. But hormonal deficiencies are a relatively rare cause of sexual problems, and focusing on hormones may distract you from more relevant underlying conditions, such as, for example, depression.

You and your partner may well be able to account for and resolve any transient sexual difficulties on your own. But if they persist or worry either of you, it is worth seeking help. A GP can listen to you and conduct a full physical examination as well as testing for other conditions and reviewing any medication that you are on.

Referral to a relevant specialist may be warranted: a gynaecologist for women, urologist for men or endocrinologist (hormone specialist) for both. But the most specific help will come from a psychosexual therapist – a therapist trained in sexual problems. You can be referred by your GP or through the organisation Relate,★ and help is available on the NHS. A list of sexual and relationships clinics can also be obtained from the British Association of Sexual and Marital Therapy.★

Therapy techniques that can be used include:

• general counselling
• techniques derived from the sex therapists Masters and Johnson. These involve refraining from sexual intercourse for a given time

while exploring non-genital intimacy, for example cuddles. Treatment goals are agreed in advance so as to replace experiences of failure with success and anxiety with enjoyment. This usually entails practice ('homework') between sessions
- specific couple therapy, which may be necessary to treat problems with communication or to enhance a couple's skills in resolving conflict and solving problems
- highly specialised help of the sort that is required for gender identity problems and paraphilias (see below).

Glossary

Atrophic vaginitis   Sore, dry vagina, usually after menopause

Dyspareunia   Painful sex for a woman

Erectile dysfunction   Impotence. Penis does not get hard enough, or stay hard long enough, for intercourse

Libido   Sex drive

Orgasm   To climax or 'come'

Paraphilias   Sexual preferences that are unwelcome to you, others or society, e.g. sadomasochism or fetishism, including paedophilia

Psychosexual therapist/counsellor   Someone qualified to investigate and advise about sexual problems that do not have a physical basis or which have a predominantly psychological cause, e.g. premature ejaculation, vaginismus

Prostatitis   Inflammation of the prostate gland causing pain on ejaculation for a man

Transsexualism   A lifelong feeling that you were born the wrong gender

Vaginismus   Vagina too tight for intercourse, due to muscle spasm

---

Low sex drive

Q *I am 45 and my sex drive is zero. It's not that I'm lusting after anyone else, I've just gone off the whole idea of sex. Could there be any physical cause, or is it all psychological?*

A Ask yourself whether it is just sex you have gone off, or life in general; in other words, are you depressed? If you are sad, negative, not sleeping, not eating and are tired all the time, you need help for depression. If you are not depressed but very sluggish, you could have an underactive thyroid (see Chapter 1), which can be checked for with a blood test. Loss of libido can be hormonal – for example, in the run-up to the menopause – although this is a relatively rare cause. Many drugs, including alcohol, can cause loss of libido as a side-effect, so if you drink, try cutting it out for a while, and check the information leaflets of any prescription drugs you are on to see whether they are possible culprits. If they are, you could talk to your GP about stopping or changing them.

Q *Since the birth of my daughter four years ago I don't feel the same emotionally, and my sex drive has vanished. I am 25 years old and feel abnormal. I have sought professional advice and am coming towards the end of counselling and medication. Although I feel better in myself my sex drive is still non-existent and is ruining a long-term relationship. Do I need HRT of any kind, or is there any sort of test that should be carried out to determine whether I need it?*

A Many women, and some men, find their sex drive diminished after they have children. A combination of factors may contribute to this: tiredness, depression, lack of privacy or opportunity, pain or some concurrent illness, and occasionally hormonal imbalance.

You have to make more of an effort to want and to have sex once you have children. It is important to get your daughter into a night-time routine that gives you some time to wind down. You need protected time alone with your partner in a setting that allows some romance to be rekindled. You should be able to have fun with him – on a date, for example. If you are depressed, you will find it hard to enjoy anything, let alone sex.

Hormonal imbalance is rarely a major factor and is unlikely to be the cause unless your periods are very erratic, you are having hot flushes, or your vagina is sore and dry. Some women have such a horrific experience of childbirth that they need specific counselling to come to terms with it before they can enjoy sex again.

Relate★ offers sexual counselling and advice in addition to help with relationships.

Q *Some time ago I had a highly sexual love affair. Four years on, I'm back with my husband but I find sex with him repellent, although he is a good man and in many ways I am happy with him. What should I do?*

A Clearly you had no problem enjoying sex during your love affair. The implication is that it is sex with your husband that is less than satisfactory and you really need to explore that, preferably with him. You should both go to Relate,* which offers couples an excellent psychosexual counselling service.

Q *My husband and I are both in our sixties and have been married for over 40 years now. He still wants to have sex at least once a week but I just can't summon up any enthusiasm. It's not that I don't love him. I do, but not in a physical way any more. Is this unusual?*

A There are so many reasons why sex may become a less attractive proposition as we get older. Libido often, but not always, wanes as we age. After the menopause hormonal changes may make the vagina dry (atrophic vaginitis), so sex is uncomfortable and may further decrease libido. Medication – for high blood pressure or depression, for example – can affect libido. Many medical conditions affect libido: for example, diabetes can affect orgasm in both sexes, contribute to impotence in men and predispose you to thrush, which also makes the vagina sore. If you have painful joints or backache from osteoarthritis, moving around the bed can be painful, although you may be able to find sexual positions which are more comfortable.

Lifestyle can also play a part. Alcohol may loosen inhibitions in small doses but larger doses affect libido and performance. If you have become very overweight or you do not feel good about your body, you may not see yourself as a sexual being any more. It is also possible that after so many years of marriage, sex has become predictable and unexciting.

Few of these causes are irreversible. You need to talk frankly to your partner in a blame-free and relaxed way. Professional help from the organisation Relate* may help you to clarify your thoughts. Changing medication, considering HRT and treating other medical problems may all help. Joining a keep-fit class, cutting down on alcohol, stopping smoking if you do, and finding ways to make you feel better about yourself (such as a facial or new hairdo) might give you a new lease of life. You and your husband may want to spice up your sex life, for example by watching sexy videos or experimenting with different positions. Take it slowly and do not rush into intercourse until you feel ready. Kissing, touching and petting may arouse your libido and revive your interest in sex. If none of this makes a difference, you may both agree to disagree on this one and reach some compromise about other ways for your husband to find the sexual fulfilment he needs.

Fear of sex

Q *I am a woman in my late twenties. I have never had sex and am beginning to wonder if I ever will. I had a few fumbled attempts with boys of my own age when I left school but never actually had proper intercourse. When I did try, it just hurt and I felt too tense to be able to go any further. I have become too frightened of sex to be able to contemplate actually enjoying it one day. Can you help?*

A You may have a condition called vaginismus (see below). However, the main problem is likely to be that sex has acquired negative associations for you. It will take time to dissociate sex from these feelings and start associating it with pleasure. You could be helped in this by a psychosexual counsellor (available either through your GP or Relate★), although there are ways in which you can help yourself.

It is very important for you to feel totally at ease with your body and genitals. Try looking closely at your vagina and vulva with a mirror. If you do not use tampons you may not be used to inserting a foreign body into your vagina. Self-exploration with your fingers, or using a vibrator, while lying relaxed in bed will introduce you to the pleasurable sensations that you can experience in a sexual relationship with a partner.

It may be that your choice of potential partners has been wrong for you. You might feel more comfortable with an older, more sexually experienced man, or you may be more attracted to women but have not explored that idea. Penetrative, heterosexual sex is not for every woman. Finally, you may have to readjust your expectations of sex – for most women the first time is rarely enjoyable. It is often anxiety-inducing and a bit painful.

You should be free from worries about pregnancy or sexually transmitted diseases, so make sure you have a reliable form of contraception, such as the pill, and ask your partner to use a condom. A comfortable, clean, warm and private setting will enable you to feel as relaxed as possible. Alcohol helps to release inhibitions, and Vaseline or KY jelly will aid lubrication. Remember that sex, like wine and good cheese, definitely gets better with time – so do not judge your future experiences in the light of your past.

Painful sex

Q *I am experiencing pain when I have sex. I am unable to carry on after I have an orgasm as my vagina becomes too sore and tender. At first I thought this might change as I got more used to sex, but it has been going on for more than a year now. What could be causing it?*

A Pain during sex (dyspareunia) is upsetting and can trigger off a vicious cycle, because the pain makes you lose your enjoyment of sex, which in turn makes you tense up or remain dry and makes sex even more uncomfortable. Sex may be painful near the entrance of the vagina, making penetration difficult or even impossible. Common causes are:

- tense vaginal muscles (vaginismus – see below) due to anxiety about sex and insufficient stimulation and lubrication
- dry vagina due to lack of stimulation or hormonal changes, e.g. after the menopause
- inflamed vagina due to infection, e.g. thrush (see Chapter 5)
- torn or poorly-healed vagina, e.g. after childbirth.

Sometimes penetration is fine but sex becomes painful during deep thrusting. This can be caused by conditions that involve inflammation of pelvic organs, such as endometriosis, ovarian cysts, pelvic inflammatory disease (see Chapter 5 for more about these) or irritable bowel syndrome (see Chapter 7). If penetration and deep thrusting are not painful but you get sore towards the end of intercourse, it may be that you are not fully lubricated so the repeated friction is making you sore. Try using condoms which are lubricated, put some Vaseline in your vagina before sex (although if you are using condoms you must use a water-based lubricant instead), and ask your partner to withdraw once you have both reached orgasm. If soreness is still a problem, you may want to be checked for infections such as thrush (see Chapter 5), which could be inflaming your vagina.

Some women put up with painful sex for various reasons. This is not a good idea. At the very least, it prevents the woman from enjoying sex and will lead to decreased arousal and less likelihood of orgasm. At worst, she may be ignoring a problem for which treatment is available.

Q *I get terrible pain in my vagina whenever I try to have sex. I can't even bear my partner's penis to enter my vagina at all before I start to tense up with the pain. I know that he thinks this means I don't love him. I haven't had sex before although I did try once with someone else and the same thing happened. I've never been able to put anything in my vagina and can't use tampons for the same reason. I'm 26 and am worried I won't ever be able to have a sexual relationship. How can I get help?*

A You do need to grasp the nettle and make an appointment to see a sympathetic female GP or doctor at a family planning clinic. She will examine you to check there is no physical cause for your inability to have sex. This may be quite difficult for you and you might need some time before you feel comfortable enough with the doctor to have a physical examination. You will need a smear test and some swabs, if there is any discharge, as infections can be a cause of painful sex.

However, it is highly likely, from what you have said, that the real problem is vaginismus.

This is a condition whereby an involuntary spasm of the muscles surrounding the vaginal opening makes any attempt at vaginal penetration either extremely painful or altogether impossible. Most women who suffer from vaginismus are still capable of becoming sexually aroused, and achieving orgasm, through stimulation of the clitoris.

Vaginismus is generally considered to be a psychosomatic disorder – a physical manifestation of a psychological cause. This cause is likely to relate to either control issues within the sexual relationship, past sexual trauma, or a phobic reaction to the thought of penetration – i.e. an association of pain or fear with vaginal penetration.

A psychosexual counsellor – available through your GP or the organisation Relate* – will be able to help. Treatment usually involves a combination of couples therapy, prescribed Kegel exercises (for the pelvic floor muscles) or sensate focus exercises (a technique for couples to become reacquainted sexually, by focusing initially on non-sexual sensuality) for you and your partner to do at home, and the progressive use of a plastic dilator or finger (yours or your partner's), inserted into the opening of your vagina to gradually stretch the contracted muscles.

The cure rate for vaginismus when treated by a professional using these, or similar, techniques is very high. A significant factor in whether the treatment is successful, however, is the support you have in coping with the anxiety which will almost inevitably arise from knowing that being cured will mean allowing the penetration which you fear. Ideally, this anxiety will be confronted and dealt with in the couples therapy.

Q *During sex, my cervix often feels sore and deep penetration can be quite painful. Is this due to lack of lubrication or something more serious? Often if I shift position, it improves. I was once told by a doctor that I have a retroverted uterus – is this the cause of the problem?*

A A retroverted uterus is one that tips backwards rather than forwards. It may cause some discomfort during particularly deep penetration but would not usually cause any soreness of the cervix.

Many women sometimes feel discomfort or pain with deep penetration. This may be a normal response to the pressure on sensitive internal parts. You can exercise some control over the depth of penetration by adopting different positions, such as:

- woman on top, controlling the depth of penetration
- woman on her back, with her legs flat, or one leg flat and one pulled back
- woman on her back with her legs together (usually the woman must have her legs apart to allow the man to enter; then she puts her legs together, with his on the outside of hers).

If this problem persists, you should consult your GP or ask for referral to a gynaecologist. It could be a sign of infection, including a sexually transmitted disease (see later in this chapter), a bladder infection or a condition such as endometriosis (see Chapter 5).

It is possible that your soreness is due to a cervical erosion. This is a very common cause of bleeding between periods and after sex, and is absolutely nothing to worry about. It refers to a raw area on the neck of the womb (cervix) and is not actually an erosion at all. The cervix has tough cells that line the surface which is in contact with the vagina, and delicate cells that line the inner surface of the cervix. The hormones of pregnancy and the contraceptive pill can encourage the delicate cells to grow round on to the surface in contact with the vagina. These delicate cells tend to bleed when they come into contact with tampons or the penis during sex, and can cause discomfort.

An erosion usually clears up on its own once the pregnancy ends or the pill is stopped. If troublesome, it can be easily and painlessly cauterised by touching it with a silver nitrate-tipped stick. GPs and gynaecologists can do this and no anaesthetic is necessary. It does not hurt and almost always does the trick. A smear test can be done at the same time, if it is due, and swabs taken if there is any sign of infection which may be contributing to the problem.

Q *Recently I have been suffering from pain when I ejaculate. My GP said I have prostatitis and gave me antibiotics. Can you tell me how serious this is?*

A Prostatitis is a fairly common condition causing inflammation of the prostate gland. It usually affects men aged 30–60 and causes a strong urge to urinate frequently, pain during urination and ejaculation, and generalised pelvic pain in, around and above the penis and deep inside the anus.

It is likely that you have a one-off bout of prostatitis (acute bacterial prostatitis) caused by a urinary tract infection in which the bugs from the bladder get into the prostate. Antibiotics are effective in clearing it up. If you have frequent urinary tract infections or your immunity is impaired, you may get several bouts of prostatitis (chronic bacterial prostatitis), which is quite rare. Seeing a urologist who specialises in prostatitis will allow you to discuss treatment options. See Chapter 4 for more information about pelvic pain, prostatitis and other prostate problems.

Dissatisfying sex

Q *Can a woman be impotent? I feel sexy, but when my partner and I have intercourse I very rarely reach orgasm. Although my partner does everything I tell him and we are very happy together, this does affect our relationship. I quite often end up crying after sex.*

A It is common, but not often acknowledged, that many women do not gain as much sexual satisfaction from intercourse as they would like and do not reach orgasm. It helps if you can tell your partner when he does something that particularly stimulates you, and let him know what you find a turn-off.

Certain drugs, such as drugs to lower blood pressure and most antidepressants, can interfere with your sexual enjoyment, so if you are on any medication at all you could discuss with your GP whether it can affect sex drive and whether there are alternatives. If you are run down or tired, you are unlikely to enjoy sex as much as if you are in perfect physical health. So you may want to look at your lifestyle and perhaps have a health check-up, including blood tests for anaemia, if you are particularly tired.

Your state of mind obviously influences how you feel about sex, so if you are depressed or very anxious, this may be manifesting itself in bed. You also need to ask yourself whether you have felt more sexual pleasure with other partners than your current one, and whether your feelings about sex with him are a reflection of how you feel about him rather than any lack of sex drive in you. Finally, sex drive and the ability to reach orgasm may occasionally be due to hormonal fluctuations – some women approaching the menopause rediscover their ability to enjoy sex once they start HRT; others find that changing their contraceptive pill can alter their sex drive. It is worth discussing this with your GP initially, and asking for referral to a psychosexual counsellor, either via the GP or through the organisation Relate,★ if the problem persists.

Q *I have had one or two sexual relationships before my current boyfriend, but for me sex has never been the ecstatic experience that it seems to be for most people. I don't find it painful but I am usually left feeling a bit disappointed, and I have never had an orgasm. Is there anything wrong with me, and is there anything I can do about it?*

A You may be reassured to know that you are certainly not alone in your feelings. According to the American Urological Association, lack of enjoyment of sex, and failing to have an orgasm, is the most common complaint among the 43 per cent of (American) women who have some type of sexual 'problem'. This is often the result of not having enough experience or not experimenting with what makes you happy. You may also find that the constant diet of sex in magazines puts pressure on you and raises your expectations.

Sexual inadequacies sometimes mirror more complex problems within the relationship with your partner and it may be worthwhile focusing on that. Your experience of sex may be marred by previous bad experiences or even childhood sexual abuse, which you need to talk about and work through.

Most of us shy away from the idea of seeking expert help for such an intimate and private matter. But in the UK three organisations train people to offer discreet, common-sense-based and non-intrusive help which really could make a difference to your sexual life. Therapists registered with the Institute of Psychosexual Medicine,★ the British Association of Sexual and Marital Therapy★ and Relate★ will all be bona fide and well trained, so you could approach one of them.

The Institute of Psychosexual Medicine trains doctors to offer simple psychotherapy aimed at giving women 'permission' to enjoy their own body, including their breasts, clitoris and vagina. A vaginal examination by the doctor offers reassurance about their normality and often allows women to open up about their fears.

Relate's therapists tend to work with couples to explore the psychological problems getting in the way of a fulfilling sex life. You will usually be encouraged to refrain from intercourse while concentrating on sessions in which your partner strokes and touches you. This is known as 'sensate focus' and is based on work by Americans Masters and Johnson in the 1960s.

There have been attempts to treat women with lack of sex drive or inability to reach orgasm with hormones such as the male hormone, testosterone, but they have been largely abandoned as being potentially dangerous and rarely effective. Sildenafil (Viagra) has been shown in some small studies to increase clitoral blood flow and enhance the sexual enjoyment of women after the menopause but results are less convincing for pre-menopausal women and it is not yet licensed for use by women. A vacuum pump that can be fitted over the clitoris to increase blood flow to it has been tested in women and is now licensed in the USA for women who experience reduced sensation and lubrication and an inability to reach orgasm. Known as the Eros clitoral therapy, it is likely to make its way to the UK soon. With nearly half of all women reporting lack of sexual fulfilment, the push to develop drugs or techniques that help is huge and the chances of there being a female version of Viagra within a few years is very high indeed.

Premature ejaculation

Q *After my wife died I was not sexually active for many years, but I have now found a new partner with whom I have developed a loving relationship. We would like to be able to make love but the first couple of times we tried, I ejaculated very quickly. I am rather upset by this, when things are otherwise going so well, and need advice. What should I do?*

A It is entirely natural that after many years of abstinence, you will feel that you are ejaculating quicker than you would like. This is likely to improve if you continue having sex regularly. A quick-fix solution is to take a small dose of an antidepressant (e.g. paroxetine, Seroxat, 20–40mg), 4–6 hours before intercourse. This improves the average time that a man can maintain his erect penis inside the vagina without ejaculating from less than one minute to over two minutes in half of all cases. Response is unpredictable; some men have a modest improvement, others can go as long as eight or nine minutes after taking an antidepressant. However, you will need to see your doctor to discuss this and need to bear in mind that all pills have potential side-effects. The best advice is probably to do nothing: with a bit of mutual understanding, the problem will probably solve itself.

Q *What can I do about premature ejaculation? When I make love to my girlfriend I come so quickly that she is frustrated. This is having a serious effect on our relationship. Can you suggest anything?*

A Premature ejaculation is one of the most common male sexual problems, although it is difficult to define precisely. Some 75 per cent of all men who have sex are said to ejaculate within two minutes of putting their penis inside a vagina – but ejaculation can be considered to be 'premature' if either partner is troubled by it. The embarrassment and stigma associated with premature ejaculation can affect men's sexual self-confidence – which may contribute further to the problem – to the extent, in some cases, of putting them off relationships altogether.

Although some research suggests that premature ejaculation may be, at least partially, a medical disorder, most explanations involve psychological factors. These include the following.

- **Experiences of sex while growing up**. You may have learned to 'come' quickly because it was something to be ashamed of, perhaps while masturbating at school. This can be hard to unlearn even when you no longer have to hurry.
- **Fear of not being sexually stimulated enough**. You may not be very turned on or ready for sex, despite getting an erection. You come quickly and a bit half-heartedly, whereas if you were more excited, you could wait longer and enjoy your orgasm more.
- **Fear of failure**. The more you worry about premature ejaculation or sexual performance in general, the more likely you are to come too quickly or be unable to get an erection at all. Deciding not to even attempt intercourse for a while is often the best way to take the heat off you until you feel more confident within the relationship and about your sexual performance.

These are some helpful methods which a psychosexual counsellor may discuss with you.

- **Changing position of lovemaking**. The missionary position may make you come less quickly than positions that generate more friction (e.g. woman on top). You may also be able to train yourself not to thrust as deeply at first.
- **Start-stop and squeeze techniques**. You and your partner are given a series of exercises to increase the length of time you can hang on without coming. In the squeeze technique, you or your partner squeezes the end of you penis and counts to ten when you feel like coming.
- **Psychological programming**. Although thinking about work during lovemaking is a turn-off, thinking about calming, pleasant thoughts may slow you down without turning you off.

- **Drugs**. Two antidepressants, fluoxetine (Prozac) and clomipramine (Anafranil) have both been shown to help a high percentage of men worried by premature ejaculation.

Impotence

Q *I have been impotent for many years. I have never had the courage to overcome my embarrassment and go to a doctor about it. Could there be any medical cause of my problem, and is there really any treatment that could help me after all this time?*

A It is such a shame that you have not felt able to seek help until now, because there is so much that can be done to restore your erections and enable you to have an active sex life.

Impotence, or 'erectile dysfunction', refers to an inability to get an erection or maintain one for long enough to have sex. Virtually every man experiences this at some time in his life, although it is usually a temporary response to factors such as stress or drinking too much alcohol. However, for many men impotence is a consistent problem. It is often due to psychological factors – most men with impotence still get erections at night or first thing in the morning – and long-term impotence will almost certainly have a psychological effect on a man, whatever its original cause.

Sometimes men assume that erectile problems are a natural consequence of ageing, and it is true that as you get older it may take a bit longer to get aroused or more stimulation to maintain an erection. However, the main reason that erectile dysfunction is more common among older men is that they are more likely to have medical conditions, or be taking medication, that cause impotence. Many cases of impotence are linked to physical conditions or their medication, and it is important to seek medical help for the problem, if only in order to eliminate any underlying physical cause. These include:

- disorders that affect the blood vessels and restrict blood flow to the penis, such as diabetes, heart disease, high blood pressure or high cholesterol (see Chapter 1)
- conditions that interrupt the normal connection between the central nervous system and the penis, such as prostate surgery, traumatic injury, multiple sclerosis or Parkinson's disease
- depression (see Chapter 2)

- medications (including some used to treat high blood pressure and depression) that bring about impotence as an unwanted side-effect.

The major types of prescription drugs that can cause impotence include:

- oestrogens – used in the treatment of prostate cancer
- diuretics – used for men with heart disease and hypertension
- methyldopa (Aldomet) – an older treatment for blood pressure
- beta-blockers – used in the treatment of heart disease and hypertension
- calcium channel blockers – treatments for hypertension
- tranquillisers
- decongestants
- seizure medications
- drugs to lower cholesterol
- cimetidine (Tagamet) – a drug for ulcers
- digoxin (Lanoxin) – a drug for heart failure.

'Recreational' drugs are also a major cause of erectile dysfunction – the major one being tobacco. Experiments show that even two cigarettes, if smoked before sex, will markedly decrease the blood flow to the penis. Cannabis and alcohol are big culprits too. Chronic alcoholism can cause damage to the testicles and the loss of testosterone.

The first step in treating impotence is to identify and treat any underlying physical cause or change any medication that may be contributing to it. If no such cause is found, there are various medical options available, as detailed below. Treatment for impotence has been revolutionised by the tablet sildenafil (Viagra – see below). You may also want to be referred to a psychosexual therapist (a counsellor trained in sexual problems – available via your GP or the organisation Relate★) or a urologist (a specialist in urinary and penile problems).

Most men would prefer to start their treatment by changing any medication that may be contributing to the problem, and cut down on alcohol. Taking oral drugs, such as Viagra, and going in for counselling are the next steps for most people. After that, they could go in for a range of options to aid erections which are available from impotence clinics, usually run by urologists. These include vacuum devices, drugs injected into the penis, pellets inserted into the penis, implanted devices and occasionally surgery to correct underlying disease (e.g. of blood vessels to the penis).

Viagra has revolutionised the treatment for impotence. It works by boosting the body's nitric oxide which expands blood vessels in the penis. A person taking it still needs sexual stimulation to get an erection. Viagra comes in three strengths, 25, 50 and 100mg, and it makes sense to start with the lowest dose and work your way up if needs be. You should take it one hour before sex and not more than once a day.

Another drug, the male hormone testosterone (Restandol), can be taken orally, by patch or by injection. If you have low levels of testosterone, supplementing it may help your sex drive and erections. But most men who have problems with impotence have normal levels of testosterone.

Drugs (e.g. alprostadil – Caverject) that stimulate an erection can be injected into a blood vessel in the penis and men can be taught to do this for themselves. The disadvantages of injecting such drugs are that it could be painful and men may get a persistent and painful erection (known as priapism).

Another technique is to insert a pellet of alprostadil (Caverject) into the urethra using an applicator, which is marketed under the name MUSE. It works well and is less off-putting to many men than an injection. It can make the penis ache, look red or cause some discomfort and even bleeding in the urethra.

Vacuum devices use a plastic cylinder around the penis with a pump attached which draws air out of the cylinder, creating a vacuum around the penis. This makes the penis fill up with blood, thus engorging it. You then pop an elastic band round the base of the penis to keep it that way until you have had intercourse. Your penis may look a bit odd – purplish and cylinder-shaped – but such a device is effective, and does not involve any drugs, injections or pellets.

Surgery can be used to implant a device that you can inflate when you need an erection. But these implants may get infected or damaged and, like surgery to repair damaged blood vessels, are considered to be a last resort in the treatment of impotence.

Viagra

Q *Is it safe for me to take Viagra? I have high blood pressure and slightly high cholesterol, and have heard that this could make it dangerous.*

A A new analysis of 53 studies of men treated for erectile problems showed that those on sildenafil citrate (Viagra) had a lower risk of heart attacks and death than those taking a placebo. The guidance now is that anyone with a stable heart condition can take it without too much concern.

However, men with existing and poorly controlled conditions such as heart disease may be at greater risk. For example, Viagra should not be taken in combination with nitrate drugs for heart disease, as it increases the effect of these drugs. Your GP will be able to discuss your personal risks with you.

You should be fully checked out by your doctor and perhaps have an exercise ECG (electrocardiogram – which shows whether you have had a recent heart attack or are experiencing heart strain at present) to check that exertion does not put a strain on your heart – it is not the Viagra but sex that could be a bit much for you, so a check-up may be a reassuring step.

In general, side-effects are uncommon with Viagra, although some men may experience a headache or flushing of the skin. Occasionally, Viagra can cause a prolonged erection which becomes painful and can cause permanent damage to the penile tissue. If an erection resulting from the use of Viagra lasts longer than four hours (priapism), immediate medical treatment should be sought.

There is no evidence to suggest that using Viagra affects male fertility.

Q *My husband has been impotent for several years. His doctor has given him a prescription for Viagra without discussing what other medication he is on. Is this relevant?*

A You are right to be concerned about sildenafil citrate (Viagra) being prescribed without an opportunity to discuss the physical and psychological factors that may be contributing to your husband's impotence. It is quite possible that any medication he takes – for example, for high blood pressure – is causing the impotence and that changing the medication may be enough to restore his erections without needing to take Viagra at all. And if psychological factors are playing a part, which they almost certainly are by now even if the original cause of impotence was physical, he might well benefit from some expert psychosexual counselling, available via the GP or from the organisation Relate.★

Sexually transmitted diseases

Q *I have just embarked on my first sexual relationship and want to ensure protection against sexually transmitted diseases, especially HIV. I know that it is important to practise safe sex, but am not so sure what exactly safe sex is. Can you explain it for me?*

A The only way to be absolutely certain of never getting a sexually transmitted disease (STD) is never to have sex at all, and that would make life extremely dull. It stands to reason that the more partners you have, the more times you are exposing yourself to the possibility of infection, so restricting the number means lowering the risk. Safe sex means making sure that your partner's blood, semen and vaginal fluids do not enter your body. Infections can also be passed on through contact with open sores (e.g. herpes), and safe sex can avoid this spread. Safe sex could take the form of avoiding vaginal or anal penetration (e.g. mutual masturbation or restricting yourselves to cuddling and touching); using condoms for vaginal or anal sex; avoiding oral sex if you have open mouth ulcers or bleeding gums; and not giving your partner oral sex if you have a cold sore. Cold sores are caused by the herpes simplex virus (see page 268).

Q *Recently I had sex with someone after a party when I was drunk and we didn't use a condom. I know it was stupid and now I can't stop worrying that I may have caught a sexually transmitted disease. How will I be able to tell?*

A You may have reason to suspect you have got an STD if you have a vaginal discharge or irritation, urethral discharge (oozing from the penis), or ulcers on your genitals. You can go to your GP, a family planning clinic or an STD clinic (found in most hospitals – ring your local hospital and ask for the STD clinic), and should be offered a chance to explain your symptoms and medical history. You will be asked about your number of sexual partners, your sexual orientation (i.e. homosexual, heterosexual or bisexual), the age at which you first had sex, the type of contraception you have used, whether you have ever been pregnant or had terminations of pregnancy (abortions), and so on.

These questions may seem intrusive and irrelevant but they are supposed to be non-judgemental and they are essential to making an accurate assessment. You will certainly be examined and samples taken from your vagina or penis, and often from your anus too. Women may often be offered a cervical smear at the same time as the internal vaginal examination. Blood tests may be necessary to test for infections. If you do have an STD, it will be important to trace any sexual contacts, and you will be asked for their details. You may feel reluctant to pass on this information, but it is vital in preventing the spread of these often highly infectious diseases – and is undoubtedly in these people's interests to be contacted, as they may be harbouring an infection, such as chlamydia, that could impair their fertility if not treated.

Treatment of most STDs requires antibiotics or anti-viral medication, and the practice of safe sex – i.e. abstinence or use of condoms – until you are clear of infection.

Sexually transmitted diseases

The three most common STDs seen in UK STD clinics are genital warts, urethritis and chlamydia. Gonorrhoea still exists but is declining steadily, and syphilis is no longer a major problem. Other common sexually transmitted conditions include trichomonas, genital herpes and pubic lice. Scabies (see Chapter 9), vaginal thrush and bacterial vaginosis (BV) (see page 100 and Chapters 5 and 8) are often seen in STD clinics but are not actually sexually transmitted. (Scabies and thrush can sometimes be contracted through sexual contact but it is not essential for their transmission.) Other viruses, including hepatitis B and C, are also increasingly common, and HIV remains a serious public health concern.

Further details about each of these are given below.

Genital warts

Q *I have some small lumps on my penis that look like little warts. They are not painful, but should I get them looked at?*

A Small warty-looking lumps on the glans, shaft and foreskin of the penis are often genital warts. Also known as venereal warts, they are one of the most common types of sexually transmitted diseases. As well as being infectious to others, they are infectious to the person who has them, so what starts as a single wart can quickly become a cluster.

The warts may look like small, flesh-coloured bumps, or have a cauliflower-like appearance. Sometimes they are only one or two millimetres in diameter, but they can also multiply into clusters, which can be quite large. They affect the moist areas of the genital area. In men, they may be found on the tip or shaft of the penis, the scrotum or the anus. In women, they can grow on the vulva, the walls of the vagina, the perineum (the area between the external genitals and the anus) and the cervix (the neck of the uterus). They also can develop in the mouth or throat of a person who has had oral sexual contact with an infected person.

Genital warts are usually treated by painting on a chemical known as podophyllin (Posalfilin). You do need to get them treated, because they can infect any sexual partners that you have and can put women at increased risk of cervical cancer. There are also reports of untreated genital warts becoming malignant – i.e. cancerous.

Urethritis

Q *I have a discharge from the hole at the end of my penis, where urine and sperm come out. I'm worried sick – what could it be?*

A A urethral discharge is the most common sign, in men, of a sexually transmitted disease, although not all the causes are sexually transmitted. The possible causes are:

- sperm leaking out
- gonorrhoea
- non-gonococcal urethritis – i.e. all infectious causes that are not due to gonorrhoea. These could include chlamydia, trichomonas, candida (thrush), various bacterial infections, lumps inside the urethra (e.g. warts, herpes or syphilis), allergy (e.g. to latex) or foreign bodies (e.g. things inserted into the urethra for sexual stimulation). In 25 per cent of cases of non-gonococcal urethritis the cause is never discovered.

(See Chapter 4 for more about urethral discharge.)

Chlamydia

Q *My girlfriend has been told that she has chlamydia and has been given antibiotics. Her doctor told her to tell me to get treatment too. What is chlamydia and do I really need treatment?*

A You do need to get treatment, if only to reduce the risk of re-infecting your girlfriend and causing her to have fertility problems in the future. Chlamydia is a bacterial infection of the genital tract that spreads easily through sexual contact. The disease is not difficult to treat, but if it is left untreated it can lead to more serious health problems. Chlamydia is the most common bacterial sexually transmitted disease in the UK.

Chlamydia is difficult to detect because early-stage infections often cause few or no symptoms, and if symptoms do occur they can be mild and transient. Symptoms may occur one to three weeks after exposure to the bacterium, and could include:

• painful urination
• lower abdominal pain
• vaginal discharge in women
• discharge from the penis in men.

The other health problems that chlamydia can lead to include:

• pelvic inflammatory disease in women (see Chapter 5)
• inflammation of the epididymis, which is the tube that takes sperm from the testicle, causing fever and pain in the scrotum
• prostatitis, an infection of the prostate gland, causing pain during sex and urination (see Chapter 4)
• eye infections, if the chlamydia spreads to your eyes.

Treatment of chlamydia is with antibiotics such as erythromycin (Erymax) or doxycycline (Vibramycin).

Gonorrhoea

Q *I went to my doctor recently about some urinary problems that I have been experiencing, and was told that I have gonorrhoea. This shocked me terribly. Can you tell me more about it and how serious it is?*

A Gonorrhoea is a very infectious sexually transmitted disease, sometimes called 'the clap'. The bacterium that causes it is called

Neisseria gonorrhoeae or gonococcus. The infection develops two to ten days after you are in close sexual contact with an infected person. Gonorrhoea in men can cause a thick, pus-filled discharge from the penis, pain on passing urine or anal pain and discharge. Women often have no symptoms at all or may have a vaginal discharge, pain passing urine or a sore anus. Oral sex with an infected person can lead to gonorrhoea in the throat, but that often causes no symptoms. Untreated gonorrhoea can result in fertility problems, and the narrowing of the urethra may lead to urinary problems. Babies born to mothers infected with gonorrhoea may have inflammation of the eyes. Treatment is with antibiotics such as amoxycillin (Amoxyl) or ciprofloxacin (Ciproxin). It is essential that the course is completed otherwise resistant strains of the bacterium can emerge and long-term health problems (e.g. infertility) may result.

Syphilis

Q *I recently attended an STD clinic after I developed a discharge from my penis. They said at the clinic that one of the tests they were doing was for syphilis. I've never heard of anyone having syphilis nowadays. Is there really much chance that I could have it?*

A Syphilis is certainly much less common than it was, but it does still occur, is readily treated and can cause severe complications if left untreated.

Syphilis is a bacterial infection usually transmitted by sexual contact. The disease affects your genitals, skin and mucous membranes (e.g. the lining of the mouth, vagina and other body cavities), but may also involve many other parts of your body. It enters the body through minor cuts or abrasions in the skin or mucous membranes during sexual activity. Syphilis can also be transmitted by infected blood, and from a mother to her unborn child during pregnancy.

Signs and symptoms occur in stages. At the primary stage symptoms may occur from ten days to six weeks after exposure, and include: painless sores on the genitals, rectum, tongue or lips; enlarged lymph nodes in the groin.

At the secondary stage symptoms may begin one week to six months after the first stage, and include: rash over any area of the body, especially on palms and soles of the feet; fever; headache; soreness and aching in bones or joints.

Following the secondary stage is an intermediate period called latent syphilis. If the disease is not treated, the bacteria may spread, leading years later to the symptoms of tertiary syphilis, although this is extremely rare these days. Symptoms include: widespread infection, possibly affecting the skin, bones, brain, heart and other internal organs; blindness; psychiatric disorders; dementia.

If symptoms of the primary stage of syphilis appear, a blood test and microscopic analysis of the discharge from the open sores can confirm the presence of the bacteria. During latent syphilis, when there are no symptoms, a special blood test can diagnose the infection.

Early diagnosis and treatment with penicillin or another antibiotic can cure syphilis. After 24 hours of beginning antibiotic treatment, syphilis is no longer contagious.

Trichomonas

Q *My wife has a trichomonas infection, which was picked up on her smear test. Is it dangerous and do I need treatment?*

A Trichomonas, which is a sexually transmitted disease, causes a thin, frothy vaginal discharge with a characteristic fishy smell. Men and women who have it could suffer from discomfort when urinating though men often have no symptoms of the infection. The condition is caused by a bacterium called *Trichomonas vaginalis* (TV). The diagnosis is confirmed by growing TV from a vaginal swab. TV can be sexually transmitted and if a woman is found to have the infection her partner should be treated too. It is possible to have gonorrhoea at the same time as TV and they quite often co-exist. Treatment is with the antibiotic metronidazole (Flagyl); while being treated the patient has to avoid alcohol because it causes flushing and an unpleasant reaction with metronidazole. (See Chapter 8 for more about trichomonas.)

Herpes

Q *I have some sores on my penis that my girlfriend thinks might be herpes. How can I tell?*

A Sores on your penis could be caused by any of the following factors:

- too much friction after over-enthusiastic sex
- syphilis (see above)
- herpes

- scabies (see Chapter 9)
- tropical diseases
- widespread disease
- cancer of the penis, which is rare, affects elderly men and usually causes one isolated ulcer (see Chapter 4).

Herpes and syphilis are the most common causes of penile ulcers in the UK. Whereas syphilis is usually painless, herpes is painful and sore. The symptoms of herpes include pain and itchiness often before the ulcers appear, blisters or sores on the penis, and invisible but painful ulcers inside the urethra.

Herpes is caused by the herpes simplex virus. It can cause sores anywhere on the body, but generally type I of the virus infects the mouth (causing cold sores – see Chapter 10) and type II infects the genitals – but there is a substantial overlap, and it can be transmitted from mouth to genitals, or vice versa, through oral sex. The virus is transmitted to another person through a broken area of the skin (it will not enter through intact skin), usually from a cold sore or herpes blister, but also sometimes when no blisters are apparent. If you have antibodies to type I you will have some protection against type II, and vice versa – so, for example, having cold sores may protect you against getting genital herpes at a later stage.

Symptoms of genital herpes begin two to seven days after exposure. Itching or burning is followed by blisters and sores. In women, these erupt in the vagina or on the labia, buttocks and anus. In men, you may get blisters on the penis, scrotum, buttocks, anus and thighs. The virus remains dormant in the infected areas and periodically reactivates, causing symptoms.

The treatment is still unsatisfactory, as no one drug or treatment can cure the herpes or guarantee that it will not recur. Painkillers are effective, and sitting in a warm bath with a few tablespoons of salt added can be soothing. You may want to pass urine while in the bath if your penis is very sore. Anti-viral treatments, such as oral acyclovir (Zovirax), help in the first attack if given as early as possible in the course of the herpes. If you get six or more attacks a year, longer-term treatment is often advised. Herpes is not dangerous for men but can be damaging for women as it can affect the cervix. It can also damage an unborn child, possibly leading to brain damage, or even death, from encephalitis.

More information is available from the Herpes Viruses Association.*
(See Chapter 10 for more about cold sores.)

Pubic lice

Q *A friend of mine told me he has had pubic lice. I was wondering if I should avoid going round to his place, using his toilet and so on. Can you catch it easily, or just from having sex?*

A Pubic lice ('crabs') are lice that attach to coarse body hair and cause irritation. They are usually spread by close body contact and rarely by contact with unwashed bed linen, towels, etc. – although this is possible, as they can survive without a human host for one or two days. Sometimes people experience no symptoms, but usually the lice cause itching, often worse at night. Treatment involves applying a permethrin lotion to infested parts of the body, and one or two applications will usually kill the lice and eggs. If he has been treated and has thoroughly cleaned all his clothes and bedding, you should not be at any risk. You won't catch them from his toilet seat, but you may want to avoid sleeping over at his place or more intimate contact until you are certain that he has been properly treated.

Candida (thrush)

Q *What is candida? My girlfriend told me she has it and I wondered whether I can catch it?*

A Candida is a yeast that normally occurs in the mouth, vagina and intestines without causing any symptoms. This is not a sexually transmitted disease, but in women sex may irritate the vagina and allow candida to grow. This is often called thrush and is very common. If an overgrowth of this fungus occurs, it may produce an itchy vaginal discharge which requires anti-fungal treatment. In men, it can cause balanitis – inflammation of the head of the penis – which may also require treatment with anti-fungal cream.

(See Chapters 4 and 5 for more about thrush in men and women.)

Bacterial vaginosis (BV)

Q *My girlfriend has a vaginal infection called BV. Is it dangerous for me?*

A Bacterial vaginosis (BV) is an overgrowth of various bacteria which are normally present in the vagina – gardnerella is one bacterium which may be involved. The reason this change in the vaginal bacteria occurs is unclear, although some women develop BV soon after intercourse with a new partner. Symptoms may include irritation and vaginal discharge with an unpleasant odour. This condition is only treated in women who have symptoms. No counterpart to bacterial vaginosis occurs in men and treatment of male partners is not necessary.

(See Chapters 5 and 8 for more about BV.)

Hepatitis B

Q *A friend of mine has been told that she has hepatitis B, and that she might have caught it from having sex with someone who was infected. I am worried for her as I have heard that it can be fatal. Can you tell me more about it?*

A Hepatitis B is a virus that affects the liver. The virus is spread by blood-to-blood contact (e.g. sharing needles) or by sex (vaginal, oral or anal). People who are infected may have no symptoms at all or they may become ill with fever, nausea, dark urine or jaundice (yellow skin and eyes). After infection, most people recover, develop antibodies to the virus and cannot spread the virus to others. A few people retain the virus, become carriers, may infect others, and have an increased risk of developing liver disease. A vaccine for hepatitis B is available. It is not effective for hepatitis B carriers.

Hepatitis C

Q *How do you catch hepatitis C? I know someone who is a carrier and wonder how infectious he is.*

A Hepatitis C is another virus that affects the liver. So far there is no test to show whether the virus has completely cleared from a person's body or whether he or she remains a carrier (infectious to others). It is suspected that a greater proportion of people remain carriers than with hepatitis B. Long-term carriers may develop liver problems years after infection.

Hepatitis C is spread by blood-to-blood contact but appears to be not easily spread by sexual contact. Infection is more often due to sharing needles or from contaminated blood transfusions, although the latter is no longer a danger since all blood is now screened for hepatitis C. There is no vaccine available for hepatitis C.

HIV

Q *Can I catch HIV from oral sex? I have a new partner and am being very conscientious in insisting he use condoms when we have sex. But I wondered about oral sex.*

A The answer to your question is 'yes'. The risk after one-off oral sex is low but it has been shown that if you have oral sex with a man who is HIV positive, you could be at risk yourself. So avoid it until you know he is negative – something which can only be determined by an HIV test (see below).

HIV and AIDS

HIV (human immuno-deficiency virus) affects the immune system. Although people with HIV generally look and feel healthy, and may have no symptoms for some time, the virus slowly damages their immune systems. This means that HIV-positive people are less able to resist and recover from infections, and will eventually get infections or illnesses that do not usually affect those with healthy immune systems. A person has AIDS (acquired immune deficiency syndrome) when one of these illnesses occurs. Most people do not develop AIDS until many years after infection with HIV.

HIV is present in the blood, semen and vaginal fluids of people who are infected. A person who does not have the virus can become infected by contact with these fluids. The virus is spread by blood-to-blood contact (e.g. sharing needles) or by sex (vaginal, anal or oral). Once infected, a person remains infected, and infectious, for life. HIV is diagnosed by a blood test.

More advice is available from the National AIDS helpline.*

Q *I am thinking of having an HIV test because I am about to get married and would like to be certain that I am not HIV positive. Is this a good idea?*

A You do not need to have an HIV test unless you think you might be at risk (e.g. you inject drugs, have had sex with someone who injects drugs or with a person you think may be infected, or have had multiple sexual partners without practising safe sex). The test looks for antibodies in your blood to the HIV virus. You must realise that it can take up to three months after being exposed to the virus for these antibodies to build up sufficiently to show up in the blood test, so if you have been at risk for less than that period, the test may not show up as positive even if you have been infected and a negative result may give you false reassurance.

Having the test itself can be quite anxiety-inducing, and getting the result even more so. Ask the doctor or health professional taking your blood any questions you may have before going ahead with the test. When you go for the result, which is usually a week after the test, take someone with you. Being told that the test is positive is not a death sentence. It means that you have been infected with the HIV virus and that it is possible that you will develop AIDS. If you are HIV positive, you should always practise safe sex so you do not pass on the virus to anyone else. You will be referred to a specialist HIV unit, usually based in a hospital, for further tests and advice including whether and when you would benefit from medication. If you are HIV positive, you will want to stay as healthy as possible, looking after your diet, exercise regime and acting quickly if you catch even minor infections. Your partner and any other sexual contacts will also need to be tested if you are positive.

Further advice is available from the National AIDS helpline.*

All people who are HIV positive can infect others:

- during unsafe sex (see page 93)
- when sharing needles and syringes
- by blood transfusion
- from mother to baby at birth and by breast milk.

HIV is not spread by coughing, sneezing, sharing eating utensils, shaking hands, hugging or kissing.

If you are concerned about confidentiality, be careful whom you tell about having the test, or the test results. Staff at the clinic will not tell your results to anyone outside the clinic.

Apart from your health, there are other ways in which a positive result may affect you. Some insurance companies require an HIV test or disclosure of risk factors before accepting a policy. Some overseas embassies require an HIV test or declaration of any infectious diseases before issuing a visa.

Homosexuality

Q *I am 13 years old and I think I might be gay. I have got some good mates at school but I wouldn't be able to talk to them about this, and I don't think my mum and dad would like it either. What should I do?*

A Many teenagers are confused about their sexuality, so the first thing to remember is that you are not alone and certainly not the first to have such concerns. Nevertheless, it is clearly a difficult time for you, and you need to get some information and talk through your worries with a caring adult who is not personally involved with you: your GP, a counsellor at school, or a teacher perhaps. You would also benefit from reading 'A beginner's guide to coming out' on the Channel 4 web site.★

Transsexualism

Q *I have been dressing in women's clothes for many years now. For a long time I kept it completely secret but recently I told my wife, who was a bit shocked but has been supportive and sympathetic. However, I have since started feeling that I want to express this side of myself more strongly and become more physically feminine. Can you offer any advice?*

A Many men practise some form of cross-dressing and enjoy wearing women's clothes. They remain heterosexual and their cross-dressing does not usually interfere with their sexual relationship with their partner – in some cases, it provides sexual interest for both the man and woman, and some women even enjoy helping their partner to find clothes and accessories.

It is less common for men to be transsexuals – to feel that they were born the wrong gender. Transsexualism is different from cross-dressing and not to be confused with homosexuality. A transsexual man will want to dress as a woman as a natural response to his desire to become a woman.

Sex-change surgery is possible, but before a man is considered for surgery he will usually have to demonstrate that he has been successfully living as a woman for at least two years. A psychiatrist will check that there is no significant mental disorder, such as schizophrenia. The man will then be referred to a gender reassignment programme, which includes counselling on dress and behaviour in addition to female sex hormone therapy. A gender reassignment service is available at many major hospitals.

The surgery itself involves removal of the penis and testicles and construction of a vagina and breasts. This surgery is not only physically traumatic, bringing permanent infertility and impotence, but can also cause considerable psychological and psychosexual trauma. However, this risk is reduced by extensive counselling, as part of the programme, and many transsexuals find peace of mind for the first time in their lives once the transformation has been achieved.

If you are moving from cross-dressing to wondering whether you are indeed a transsexual, you need to talk to a specialised counsellor. Relate★ have well-trained psychosexual counsellors who may be helpful. You will almost certainly want to involve your wife in the counselling also.

For further advice contact the Beaumont Trust,★ which aims to support transsexuals, transvestites, and their families and friends.

Sexual deviation

Q *When I first got together with my boyfriend we were happy and our sex life was good. But then it all started to change. He wants me to do things that I don't want to do, things that seem quite perverted. A couple of times I have gone along with it to try and please him, but it made me feel dirty. Now I am starting to feel threatened and want to get out of the relationship. I still care about him enough to want to help him but I don't know how to. What should I do?*

A It is very distressing when a relationship changes such that you are drawn into a situation in which you no longer feel comfortable. You must not feel pressurised into any activity, sexual or otherwise, that pushes the boundaries of your own personal morality, pleasure or comfort.

Ideas of what is 'normal' sexual behaviour vary considerably, and may be determined by your age, cultural background, personality and previous experiences. One person's sexual deviation may be another's norm. For example, anal sex is anathema to some but is practised by 13 per cent of sexually active women in the UK and is obviously the standard in male homosexual intercourse.

Sexual deviation is a term used for sexual behaviour that goes beyond whatever is deemed socially acceptable in the age and culture in which we live. It implies a range of sexual practices that do not necessarily enhance a loving relationship. It is argued sometimes that what goes on between two consenting adults is their business alone, but in many cases of sexual deviation one partner preys on the other, who may be vulnerable and weak and unable to assert his- or herself and refuse to take part in the practices. Sexual deviation is often practised by people who have been sexually abused in childhood or who have underlying personality problems or crises involving their sexual identity. Men are more prone to sexual deviancy than women, but women do initiate and, more often, take part in sexual deviancy, so it would be wrong to think of this as a solely male problem.

Examples of sexual deviation include:

- **flashing** the exposing of the penis to (and sometimes masturbating in front of) unsuspecting women gives 'flashers' sexual excitement. Flashers rarely interfere with women and are usually harmless though upsetting
- **voyeurism** the act of watching others getting undressed or having sex. A voyeur often masturbates to relieve his own sexual excitement while watching others
- **sadism** sexual arousal from inflicting pain on others
- **masochism** sexual arousal as a result of having pain inflicted on oneself
- **bestiality** sexual activity with animals. This is illegal and can never involve bilateral consent
- **frottage** arousal from rubbing one's genitals against others in a crowd, often experienced in crowded trains and buses
- **urophilia** sexual pleasure from being urinated on
- **coprophilia** sexual pleasure from being defecated on
- **paedophilia** sexual activity involving children. This is illegal and cannot involve informed consent by a child.

It is important that you do not feel responsible for your boyfriend's behaviour. If you want to 'help' him, you could ask him to see a counsellor. Counselling that aims to discover the underlying causes of deviancy, and behaviour modification to substitute the deviant practices with less harmful ones, can be very successful if the individual is motivated to change. If you are being threatened or abused by him, contact the Rape Crisis Federation.★

Chapter 4

The male body

While most men are aware of the basic anatomy of their genitals, certainly of the visible parts, there is a great deal of ignorance about what goes on beneath the surface. Despite an increasingly open attitude towards health issues, the male genitalia remain a subject that people are reluctant to discuss seriously; indeed this is perhaps one of the last taboos. Doctors' surgeries may feature posters promoting awareness of health issues particular to women, but rarely the equivalent for men. Even worse, a jocular 'locker room' attitude still prevails among many groups of men, fostering myths and misinformation which can lead to anxiety and an unwillingness to seek medical help for a problem.

The penis is as susceptible to ailments as any other part of the body. Spots, lumps, rashes, discharges and pain are not uncommon and the cause is usually minor. It is unnecessary to suffer worry and distress, since most complaints are eminently treatable. Men who have conditions that cause an abnormality of the penis – for example, causing it to bend severely – may suffer in silence without realising that it can be cured.

Testicular cancer is the most common cancer in young men in the UK, and prostate problems are common in men over 50. It is important, therefore, that men of all ages are familiar with their own bodies so they can be aware of any changes. They should know, for example, what the signs of an enlarged prostate are, and how to examine their own testicles.

This chapter offers advice about all these symptoms and conditions, and also covers male breasts and the male 'menopause'.

Some of the symptoms referred to may be indications of a sexually transmitted disease (STD). For more on this subject, see Chapter 3.

Glossary

Circumcision   Surgical removal of the foreskin

Ejaculation   Emission of semen from the penis; usually associated with sexual stimulation

Epididymis   Tube lying behind the testicles, in which sperm are stored prior to ejaculation

Foreskin   Loose fold of skin, also called the prepuce, covering the glans in uncircumcised men

Glans   Head of the penis, covered by foreskin in uncircumcised men

Prostate   Small gland at the base of the bladder, which produces fluids that mix with sperm to make semen

Prostatitis   Inflammation or infection of the prostate gland

Scrotum   'Bag' containing testicles and epididymis

Semen   The fluid, containing sperm, that a man ejaculates, i.e. his 'come'

Urethra   Tube running through the length of the penis that takes urine from the bladder, and along which semen travels for ejaculation

Urologist   Specialist in urinary problems and (in men) penile problems

Itchy groin

Q *I have developed an uncomfortable itching in my crotch and wondered whether it might be 'jock itch'. What is this exactly? I've heard members of my gym discussing it but haven't been able to find it in any health book.*

A The charmingly named 'jock itch' is also known as 'scrot rot' or, more politely, 'thrush'.

Sore, itchy, red skin in the groin creases is often due to thrush. This is a fungal infection caused by *Candida albicans*. It thrives in hot, damp places such as the groin. To treat thrush and avoid recurrences, keep the groin area as dry and cool as possible. Dry carefully after a shower or swimming, wear loose underpants and avoid synthetic trousers or sportswear that may trap sweat.

Antifungal treatments such as clotrimazole (Canesten) cream, which is available over the counter, help to clear thrush within a few days. Recurrent or persistent thrush may be a sign of diabetes (see Chapter 1), so it is a good idea to ask your GP for a urine or blood test to check for this.

Penis

Rash on the penis

Q *After a recent period of intense work-related stress, I have developed a rash on the lower shaft of my penis along with tingling in the penis and soreness in the scrotum. I am a happily married man and can't imagine where I could have caught a disease from, if that's what it is. What could it be?*

A It may be genital herpes, which causes tiny clusters of blisters, often heralded by burning or stinging of the skin, swollen glands in the groin and feeling unwell. Persistent pain after the blisters have healed is fairly unusual and you may want to try some lignocaine gel, which is a local anaesthetic, to numb the discomfort.

If it is herpes, it may have been your first ever attack, or a recurrence triggered by stress and being run down. You could have caught herpes from your wife during oral sex even if she did not have a cold sore at the time, because the virus can persist in the vagina or mouth even if no blisters are apparent.

This does not mean that either of you have necessarily been 'playing away'. If you have never had genital herpes, you can have a blood test to check whether you have antibodies to both types of the herpes simplex virus. For your wife, this is important if you are planning a pregnancy, because it is potentially dangerous for the baby to be delivered vaginally if the mother is having a first ever attack of genital herpes, but if she has antibodies in her bloodstream it means she has already been exposed to the virus and is not at risk of a first attack. (A first attack is much more dangerous than a recurrence because known sufferers can seek treatment immediately when they get the tell-tale signs.)

You need to ask your GP to refer you to a specialist genitourinary or sexually transmitted diseases clinic so you can discuss these issues. You can get more information from the Herpes Viruses Association.★

(See Chapter 3 for more about genital herpes.)

Q *I keep getting a nasty, red, blotchy irritation on the end of my penis. It itches and feels uncomfortable. What could it be?*

A It sounds like balanitis, which is an inflammation of the head of the penis (glans). Balanitis is not sexually transmitted – it results from an overgrowth of organisms which are normally present on the skin of the glans. The condition occurs most often in men who have a foreskin (i.e. have not been circumcised). The environment under the foreskin is warm and moist, which favours the growth of the organisms that cause balanitis, especially if moisture is allowed to persist for a while. This may occur if you have not washed for a couple of days, or sometimes after sexual activity (vaginal, oral or anal – with or without a condom).

One of the most common organisms associated with balanitis is a yeast known as *Candida albicans*. Candida can cause vaginal thrush in women; therefore balanitis in men is sometimes called thrush. However, candida is normally present in both men and women, and a man will not usually develop balanitis if he has intercourse with a woman with thrush. Medication is rarely necessary, although you may want to try an antifungal cream such as clotrimazole (Canesten), but this is usually less effective than hygiene measures. The aim is to make it difficult for organisms to grow under the foreskin by keeping the area clean and dry.

Spots on the penis

Q *I have little white things just at the bottom of the head of my penis. They aren't sore or itchy in any way, but I have had them for a long time and they are starting to worry me now. What is causing them and how can they be treated?*

A It could be thrush (see above), which can cause small white patches that adhere to the penis, or the spots may just be normal glands that produce some of the secretions that keep the skin covering the penis from drying out. If you think it might be thrush, you could rub on some clotrimazole (Canesten) cream, which is available over the counter, three times a day for five days. If it is thrush the spots should clear up, and if not you won't have done any harm. If the spots persist, it is a good idea to get them checked out by your GP. Alternatively, you can pop in to a sexually transmitted diseases clinic, where they are expert at diagnosing spots, bumps and discharges on and from the penis. Your symptoms are very unlikely to indicate anything harmful or even abnormal, but for painful symptoms or blisters it is useful to make sure you do not have herpes (see page 109) or genital warts (see Chapter 3).

Lumps on the penis

Q *I have found a lump on my penis, under the foreskin, and am terrified it could be cancer. How likely is this, and what else could it be?*

A Penile cancer is a rare cause of a growth on the penis. It tends to affect older men and is extremely unusual in men below the age of 45. It is also less common among circumcised men. Symptoms could include a lump or sore, bleeding, abnormal discharge, change in skin texture or pain, and you should see a doctor if you experience any of these. The doctor will examine the penis and if there are any lumps, a small sample of tissue will be taken and examined for any cancer cells.

A cancer may be hidden under the foreskin and can spread to lymph nodes in the groin. The treatment involves radiotherapy (using X-rays or other high-energy rays to kill cancer cells and shrink tumours), chemotherapy (using drugs to kill the cancer cells) or surgery. Surgery is the most common treatment, and the amount of tissue removed depends on how advanced the cancer is.

However, lumps on the penis are much more likely to be genital warts (see Chapter 3), although they can also be caused by thickening owing to Peyronie's disease (see page 116). Some skin conditions, for example Bowen's disease (see below), which causes scaly, red-brown patches on the penis, may be pre-cancerous and need to be sampled and kept under observation.

Painful penis

Q *My penis is painful. I sometimes have a mild pain when I ejaculate, though otherwise can still enjoy sex, and at times it is uncomfortable to wee and I find I am doing so more often than usual. I have had urine and blood* *tests, a rectal ultrasound of my prostate, which was horrible, and a battery of tests for sexually transmitted infections. Every single test has proved negative. I think my GPs are sick to death of me, but I'm in despair. No one can tell me what's wrong and my penis still hurts. Where do I go from here?*

A You would be amazed how many men are walking around with so-called chronic pelvic pain syndrome, like yourself. The pain is long lasting and can be in the penis, anus or area in between. Mild urinary discomfort and pain while ejaculating are typical symptoms. Chronic pelvic pain often seems to start after you have had severe pain from an infection, operation or accident. The pain causes anxiety and that may fuel the long-term problem. Some men may be more susceptible than others, perhaps because of particularly sensitive pelvic floor muscles or a tendency for urine to reflux into the prostate gland, causing inflammation.

As in your case, in 95 per cent of cases all tests prove negative – the other 5 per cent prove to have infections in the prostate gland or bladder, which can be treated with antibiotics. The standard test to look for infection in the prostate involves a doctor putting a finger in your back passage and massaging your prostate gland until the prostatic fluids are discharged, which are then examined for bugs. However, this test is falling out of favour – not because it is revolting, but because it is considered to be unreliable.

Treatment is difficult, as you have found. Avoid activities that make the pain worse, such as cycling, for example. Hot baths are soothing, and it is thought that regular ejaculation is good because it can reduce the inflammation. Antibiotics, for example doxycycline (Vibramycin), are often prescribed for a month at a time and can be repeated if helpful. Finasteride (Proscar), a drug that shrinks enlarged prostates, looks promising. Painkillers, antidepressants and counselling to deal with the pain and anxiety can help. A large research project on chronic pelvic pain is under way in the USA, so there is hope for progress on this subject.

Bowen's disease

Bowen's disease is a skin condition which can affect middle-aged and elderly men, and which may be pre-cancerous and can develop into cancer over the years. Dermatologists usually recommend cutting the affected area out to prevent development of cancer. It is often confused with a patch of eczema and can affect the skin on the limbs as well as the penis. When it affects the penis, it is known as erythroplasia of Queyrat. There is some suggestion that it may be associated with exposure to sheep dip, weed killers and some industrial chemicals.

Discharge from the penis

Q *I have a yellowish, clear discharge from the tip of my penis. I'm a bit embarrassed to see my GP about this. What should I do?*

A You should take yourself to the nearest sexually transmitted diseases (STD) clinic – usually attached to your local hospital. A discharge from the hole at the end of your penis is called a urethral discharge and is the commonest sign, in men, of a sexually transmitted infection. Sometimes the fluid you can see is a normal body fluid such as semen. Often, however, it represents infection such as chlamydia or gonorrhoea, which you will pass on to any sexual partner. If your partner is female, her fertility may be affected and both male and female partners may develop unpleasant symptoms such as pain and discharge if you infect them. The discharge may not be due to an STD – thrush and allergies (for example to condoms) can also cause irritation and discharge.

At the STD clinic you will be offered blood, urine and penile and rectal tests to determine the cause of your discharge. You will be given treatment, such as antibiotics for gonorrhoea or chlamydia, asked to refrain from sex until the treatment is finished (usually up to three weeks) and asked for details of any people with whom you have had sex so they can be contacted and offered testing too.

Blood in semen

Q *I use a condom when making love and was recently horrified to find blood mixed with my semen when I removed the condom after intercourse. Could this be just because our sex was more lively than usual, or is it something serious?*

A Finding blood in your semen when you ejaculate is alarming but it is usually not serious and will generally get better on its own without specific treatment. It is not caused by having too much sex or trying adventurous positions. The cause may be inflammation of the prostate, small stones (made of calcium, oxalates or uric acid, which crystallise out of the urine) in the bladder, prostate or tubes that lead to them, inflammation of the testicles and tubes above them (epididymo-orchitis), sexually transmitted infections or (rarely) TB. It is very unlikely that the bleeding is caused by cancer, but if it persists for more than a few days or keeps recurring, it would be worth having tests for infections and cancers.

Bleeding is fairly common after operations such as prostate surgery. Non-cancerous growths (e.g. polyps) and cancerous lumps in the prostate, testicles or their attached tubes can also cause blood in the semen. Drugs that thin the blood, such as warfarin, and conditions that cause easy bleeding can be underlying problems. Tests and treatment depend on the likely cause and are usually undertaken by a GP and/or urologist.

(See later in this chapter for more about the prostate.)

Tight foreskin

Q *My six-year-old son has a very tight foreskin which he can't easily pull back. My husband thinks he needs to be circumcised but I am reluctant to put him through that if he doesn't need it. He doesn't seem to have any problems with passing urine. Should I be worried about it?*

A Lots of boys have tight foreskins (a condition known as phimosis) that can't be pulled back easily over the glans. No action needs to be taken so long as your son is not getting recurrent infections (balanitis). Sometimes the tightness causes the foreskin to balloon out when the boy is passing urine, but that still does not necessarily mean he needs circumcision. In 95 per cent of cases, the foreskin becomes easier to pull back (retractile) during puberty when the hormone testosterone takes effect and the penis grows bigger.

Circumcision is an operation in which part or all of the foreskin is removed. In some countries this is performed on many baby boys soon after they are born. Circumcision may be done for religious or cultural reasons, as well as in cases of phimosis or recurrent balanitis. If the operation is performed in adulthood, the patient will need a general anaesthetic. Possible complications include pain, bleeding, infection, and narrowing of the urethral opening, making urination difficult. There is a body of opinion, most vociferous in the USA, that says that circumcision decreases sexual sensation and enjoyment, although this is denied by proponents of the practice.

Adults can develop a tight foreskin in a condition called balanitis xerotica obliterans, which often appears for the first time among men in their fifties. Irregular, flat, ivory-coloured patches appear on the foreskin and glans. The foreskin becomes thickened and the opening may become narrowed. Circumcision may help to prevent the narrowing but does not always solve the problem, and some men may still need to use a dilator or catheter to open up the narrowed opening themselves.

Penis size

Q *I am sure my penis is smaller than most men's. My wife says that I satisfy her sexually but it still bothers me. I have heard that there is a penis enlargement operation but don't know anything about it. Can you tell me what is involved?*

A Many men share your anxiety but it usually indicates a more general worry about sex rather than the fact that your penis is actually particularly small or narrow. If you are sure that your wife is happy with your sexual relationship, it may be that you need to examine your feelings about sex before you consider major, dangerous and potentially unsuccessful surgery. You can do this by talking to a skilled psychosexual counsellor (available through the organisation Relate★). You could also ask your GP to examine you to reassure you that you are 'normal'.

It may help you to know that the average length of the erect male penis is 5¼ inches. Penises that are on the smaller size when non-erect tend to increase more when they become erect than a penis that looks bigger when flaccid.

There are two surgical procedures to enlarge the penis. One is to cut the suspensory ligament: this gives the appearance of a longer penis but does not actually increase its length. It also makes the penis more unstable during intercourse, and eventually more susceptible to injury. The other method is by liposuction of tissue from one part of the body which is then injected around the penis, creating a fat, wide penis but not a longer one. These procedures are not recommended and have very high complication rates. Serious side-effects include pain, infection, bleeding and lumpiness of the penis. It is not a procedure that is offered on the NHS in the UK, and few reputable urology surgeons would be willing to perform these operations.

Bent penis

Q *I have a problem that I don't really want to speak to the doctor about. My penis has always been a bit bent when erect, but over the last couple of years it has got worse to the extent that sex hurts. This is obviously a serious concern. What can I do?*

A This condition is known as Peyronie's disease. It happens because some extra tissue tethers the penis, causing it to bend when erect. The condition affects about 1 per cent of men and develops during middle age. A painful area develops on one side of the penis, and although the pain tends to abate, the penis gradually bends towards that side. No one knows the cause, although one idea is that mild damage to the penis during sex can trigger the condition in men who are predisposed to it. The penis bends gradually for up to two years and then usually stays in that position without worsening.

A small degree of curvature does not usually matter much, but if the bent penis makes sex uncomfortable or impossible, there are two basic surgical operations which can be performed to correct the condition. You should ask your GP for referral to a urologist.

Hypospadias

Q *My sister recently had a baby boy and has been told that he has hypospadias. The doctors say that it is not serious and can be treated, but we are worried. Can you tell me more about it?*

A It is always upsetting to be told there is anything wrong with a baby, and the thought that he may need treatment – especially an operation – is scary. Hypospadias is actually the most common abnormality of the genitals that baby boys can be born with. It can run in families. The tube that carries urine from the bladder to the end of the penis (meatus) is called the urethra and it runs inside the shaft of the penis. In hypospadias, the urethra does not open at the end of the penis where it should, but anywhere along the underside of the shaft of the penis. The foreskin may also look unusual. The majority (over 90 per cent) of cases of hypospadias are mild and the opening is very close to where it should be. The only problem it causes is that as the boy grows up, he may spray urine around his feet and miss the toilet bowl more than other men do. In more severe cases, the penis may bend when erect and cause problems with both sex and urination. Surgery is generally carried out when the child is one year old. The result is usually very good and further operations are not usually necessary.

Testicles

Lumps or pain in testicles

Q *I have found a lump on one of my testicles. I know I should go to my GP and get it checked out, but I am terrified that it might be cancer and am scared of hearing the worst. What else could it be?*

A Yours is a perfectly natural reaction. We all tend to assume the worst when we feel an abnormal lump. But you will gain real reassurance only from a firm diagnosis and treatment plan.

Although testicular cancer is the most common cancer in UK men between the ages of 15 and 35, it is still rare, and it is more than likely that your lump is due to a different cause. Other conditions that can produce lumps in the testicles include:

- epididymitis, or inflammation in the tubes that store sperm
- scrotal masses, caused by cysts, other inflammations, physical injury or a hernia
- hydrocele, a soft and usually painless swelling in the scrotum, caused by a collection of watery fluid
- varicocele, or swelling in the scrotum, caused by enlarged veins

- epididymo-orchitis, an inflammation of the testicle, often due to bacterial infection or the mumps virus
- torsion, or twisting of the testicle (see below).

Some of these conditions are harmless. However, it is important that you see your doctor to determine the exact cause of your lump. Even if it is cancerous, the vast majority of testicular cancers are eminently treatable and often curable, especially if detected at an early stage – which is why it is important, particularly for adolescent boys and young men, to be aware of the symptoms and to do regular testicular self-examinations (see page 122).

The doctor will first do a physical examination and order lab tests to see if the symptoms are due to infection or another cause. You may also have an ultrasound examination. If cancer is suspected, you will have blood tests, and perhaps an operation to examine and possibly remove the diseased testicle.

It is important that you go to your doctor if you experience any pain, swelling or lumps in your testicles or groin, because there are other possible causes, apart from cancer, that require urgent treatment. Testicular torsion, for example, should be treated as an emergency. Torsion happens when the soft tissue in the testicle gets twisted, cutting off the blood supply. It rarely occurs in a normal testicle, which has descended properly into the scrotum; usually, the affected testicle is abnormal in some way. Torsion happens most commonly to boys and men aged 10 to 25, and can also happen in babies up to the age of one. The symptoms are a sudden, severe pain in the groin or lower abdomen and vomiting, and the scrotum may look swollen and bruised. The pain may start after riding a bike, lifting or straining, for example. In such a case you should go to a casualty department urgently and if doctors there agreed that torsion was possible, you would be taken straight to the operating theatre and given a general anaesthetic. The twisted testicle would be untwisted and both testes fixed into position in the scrotum with an anchoring stitch. If the twisted testicle had been irreparably damaged, it might need to be removed.

Testicular cancer

Q *I have a lump in my testicle that my doctor says might be cancerous and I have been referred to the hospital for tests. I want to know what will happen next. Can you tell me what the treatment involves?*

A Any lump felt in the scrotum is considered to be a testicular cancer until it can be proved otherwise. Occasionally, it turns out not to be a lump at all, but to be caused by torsion (see above) or swelling of a testicle due to mumps or other infections. An ultrasound scan can determine whether there really is a testicular growth. If there is, the next step is to determine whether it is cancerous or not. Blood tests to check for chemicals that rise if there is a testicular tumour are measured, and if raised, lend further weight to the diagnosis of cancer. A chest X-ray and CT (computerised tomography) scan of the abdomen can check for any spread of cancer.

If cancer is not suspected, there may be scope to sample the lump (a biopsy) and examine the cells under a microscope. If there is any doubt, you will be advised to have the testicle removed.

If cancer is suspected, you will have an operation in which the testicle will be examined and possibly removed, through an incision in the groin. If the diagnosis is unclear, a pathologist can check tissue taken from the affected testicle, during the surgery, to see if cancer cells are present. If the lump is non-cancerous, there is usually no need to remove the testicle. If the lump is a malignant tumour, the testicle will be removed and the pathologist will also determine what types of cancer cells are present. The testicles contain different types of cells, and each may develop into several types of cancer. It is important for doctors to distinguish between the different types as they develop differently, and the treatment varies for each.

If the cancer has spread to lymph nodes in the abdomen, they will also be removed.

Once this has been established, blood tests, X-rays, scans and other tests may be needed to determine whether the cancer has spread to other parts of your body. If the cancer is only in the testicle or has spread to the lymph nodes in the abdomen, the cure rate is around 95 per cent. If it has spread to other parts of the body, the cure rate is about 70 per cent. If one cancerous testicle is removed, there is a 2 to 5 per cent chance that the other will become cancerous at some point, and therefore you will probably have regular follow-up examinations with a urologist or oncologist (cancer specialist).

There are two main types of testicular cancer.

- **Seminoma** This is the most common type, representing 50 per cent of all cases. It usually affects men in their mid-thirties, and can be cured in nearly every case if discovered and treated early.

- **Nonseminoma** This is a group of cancers, the majority of which are teratomas. Teratomas occur most commonly among men in their mid-twenties, and have a 60–90 per cent cure rate, depending on the type of cells in the tumour.

Surgery may be combined with radiation therapy, chemotherapy or both; it depends on the type and stage of your cancer. Your age and overall health are also factors in choosing treatment options.

Radiation therapy uses high-dose X-rays or other high-energy radiation to kill cancer cells. Seminomas are highly sensitive to radiation therapy; nonseminomas are not.

Chemotherapy uses drugs to kill cancer cells if the cancer has spread to other parts of the body. It is usually very successful and chemotherapy treatments have made the biggest difference in reducing death from testicular cancer.

(See Chapter 1 for more about cancer.)

Q *I have been diagnosed with a malignant lump in my testicle and it is going to be removed. Will this or any subsequent treatment, like chemo, affect my fertility or my sex life?*

A Most men worry that losing one testicle will make them sterile or affect their ability to have sex. However, a remaining healthy testicle will be able to maintain your normal sexual and hormone functions. Losing both testicles would make you infertile, but you can be given male hormones to keep your sexual function essentially normal. There are currently three ways to replace testosterone: intramuscular injection, which is usually given every two weeks; patches, which are applied to the skin daily; or testosterone gel, which is rubbed into the skin daily.

After the surgical removal of a testicle, you can have an artificial testicle (prosthesis) placed inside your scrotum, which has the weight and feel of a normal testicle.

The surgical removal of lymph nodes in the abdomen will not affect your ability to achieve an erection or an orgasm. It may, however, cause sterility by interfering with ejaculation. Some men recover the ability to ejaculate without treatment, and others are helped with medication. If you undergo this surgery, ask about special techniques that may protect your ability to ejaculate.

Radiation therapy will probably not affect your ability to have sex. However, radiation does interfere with sperm production. The effect is usually temporary, and most men regain their fertility within a few months.

Chemotherapy can affect fertility, and most men will be offered the opportunity to have their sperm frozen (cryopreservation) and stored at a special facility or 'bank' for later use. However, the effect on sperm production can be temporary, and many men later regain their fertility. The fatigue caused by chemotherapy may also decrease your interest in sexual activity during the months of treatment.

If you are concerned about your ability to have children now or in the future, talk to your doctor about preserving some of your sperm before the removal of one or both testicles.

(See Chapter 6 for more about fertility.)

Q *Are there any warning signs of testicular cancer apart from a lump? Is there anything that makes people more at risk?*

A There are other signs, and you should go to your doctor if you experience any pain, swelling or lumps in your testicles or groin area. Only a small percentage of testicular cancers are painful from the outset. A lump is the most common first sign, but others include: enlargement in either testicle, a feeling of heaviness in the scrotum, a dull ache in the abdomen or groin, a sudden collection of fluid in the scrotum, pain or discomfort in a testicle or the scrotum, enlargement or tenderness of the breasts, unexplained fatigue or a general feeling of being unwell. Usually the cancer affects only one testicle.

No one knows exactly what causes testicular cancer but the following factors are related to an increased risk.

- **Undescended testicles** Men who have a testicle that never descended are at greater risk, even if the testicle has been surgically relocated to the scrotum. (See Chapter 11 for more about undescended testicles in boys.)
- **Age** Testicular cancer affects younger men, particularly those between the ages of 15 and 35. It is uncommon in children and in men over 40.
- **Race** Testicular cancer is more common in white men than black men.

Testicular self-examination

Men of all ages, starting in the mid-teenage years, should examine their testicles regularly, about once a month. This way you will become familiar with your testicles and aware of any changes that might be of concern. You should do this after a warm bath or shower, as the heat from the water relaxes your scrotum, making it easier to find anything unusual.

- Stand in front of a mirror. Look for any swelling on the skin of the scrotum.
- Examine each testicle with both hands. Place the index and middle fingers under the testicle while placing your thumbs on the top.
- Gently roll the testicle between the thumbs and fingers. Remember that the testicles are usually smooth, oval-shaped and somewhat firm. It is normal for one testicle to be slightly larger than the other. A small, firm area near the rear of the testicle is nothing to worry about. Also, the cord leading upwards from the top of the testicle (epididymis) is a normal part of the scrotum.

Prostate

Q *My GP asked me if I was having any problems with my prostate. I was ashamed to admit that I have no idea what or where my prostate is or what sort of problems I could be expecting to have. I am 76 years old and generally in good health. Can you enlighten me?*

A The prostate is a small organ about the size of a walnut. It lies below the bladder and surrounds the urethra (the tube that carries urine from the bladder). The prostate makes a fluid that becomes part of semen. Semen is the white fluid that contains sperm.

Prostate problems are common in men aged 50 and older, and most can be treated successfully without affecting sexual function. A urologist is the kind of doctor most qualified to diagnose and treat prostate problems.

You should see a doctor promptly if you have any symptoms such as:

- a frequent urge to urinate
- difficulty in urinating

- dribbling of urine
- inability to pass urine (this requires urgent medical attention).

Non-cancerous prostate problems include the following. (For details of prostate cancer see below.)

Acute bacterial prostatitis is a bacterial infection of the prostate. Any man can have a one-off bout, which is usually due to a urinary tract infection in which the bugs from the bladder get into the prostate. Symptoms include fever and chills, pain when passing urine, a strong urge to urinate frequently, pain when you ejaculate and generalised pelvic pain – in, around and above the penis, deep inside the back passage and in the lower back. Acute bacterial prostatitis can be cleared up with antibiotics, and is helped by drinking plenty of liquids.

Chronic prostatitis is a prostate infection that comes back again and again. The symptoms are similar to those of acute prostatitis although they are usually milder and there is usually no fever. However, they can be more prolonged.

Chronic prostatitis is hard to treat, although it often clears up by itself in the end. The infection may be caused by bacteria (chronic bacterial prostatitis), particularly if you are very prone to recurrent urinary tract infections or your immunity is impaired. In this case antibiotics will work. Chronic bacterial prostatitis is, however, quite rare.

Far more common is **chronic pelvic pain syndrome** (see also page 140), in which there are no bacteria in your urine or prostate but the same upsetting symptoms. The prostate gland is inflamed, probably because urine refluxes into it. Antibiotics do not usually work. In some cases, it helps to massage the prostate to release fluids. Warm baths may also help, and some say that frequent ejaculating can be beneficial. Drugs that help to shrink enlarged prostates (see below) and painkillers are worth a try.

Benign prostatic hypertrophy (BPH) is a non-malignant enlargement of the prostate, and is more common in older men. More than 50 per cent of men in their sixties have BPH, and as many as 90 per cent of those in their seventies and eighties.

An enlarged prostate may eventually obstruct the urethra and make it hard to urinate. Other common symptoms are urine dribbling and the urge to urinate often, especially at night. In rare cases, the patient is completely unable to urinate. A doctor can usually detect an enlarged prostate by rectal exam (putting a gloved finger up your back passage). The doctor may also examine the urethra, prostate and bladder using a cystoscope, an instrument that is inserted through the penis. You may also have a transrectal ultrasound, where a probe is put into your back passage to give an ultrasound picture of your prostate in order to measure it and look for signs of cancerous growth.

There are several different ways to treat BPH.

- **'Watchful waiting'** is often chosen by men who are not bothered by symptoms of BPH. They have no treatment but get regular check-ups and wait to see whether or not the condition gets worse.
- **Alpha-blockers** are drugs that help relax muscles near the prostate and may relieve symptoms. Side-effects can include headaches, and sometimes men feel dizzy, lightheaded or tired. Some common alpha blockers are doxazosin (Cardura), prazosin (Hypovase), and terazosin (Hytrin).
- **Finasteride** (**Proscar**) is a drug that inhibits the action of the male hormone testosterone, by preventing its conversion to its more active form. This can shrink the prostate. Side-effects of finasteride include declining interest in sex, problems getting an erection, and problems with ejaculation. Because it is a new drug, doctors do not know its long-term effects.
- **Surgery** is the treatment most likely to relieve BPH symptoms. However, it also has the most complications. Another option is laser treatment, which has a lower chance of complications, but the disadvantage is that tissue cannot be sent to the lab to check for cancer, as it is destroyed by the laser.

Prostate cancer

Q *My father has been told by his doctor that he may have prostate cancer, and he is due for more tests. He is 71. How serious is this type of cancer, and what are the treatment prospects?*

A Prostate cancer is currently the fourth most common cancer in the UK but is set to become the most common within the next 20 years as the proportion of elderly men in the UK increases rapidly. Over 80 per cent of cases affect men over 65.

In the early stages of prostate cancer, the disease stays in the prostate and is not life-threatening. Without treatment, cancer can spread to other parts of the body and eventually cause death. Some 40,000 men die every year in the UK from prostate cancer that has spread.

To find the cause of prostate symptoms (see previous question), the doctor takes a careful medical history and performs a physical examination. This includes a digital rectal exam, in which the doctor feels the prostate through the rectum (back passage). Hard or lumpy areas may mean that cancer is present.

If a doctor suspects prostate cancer, he or she may recommend a biopsy. This is a simple surgical procedure in which a small piece of prostate tissue is removed with a needle and examined under a microscope. If the biopsy shows prostate cancer, other tests (e.g. transrectal ultrasound – see above) are done to determine the type of treatment needed.

There are several ways to treat prostate cancer. Which is chosen depends on many factors, such as whether or not the cancer has spread beyond the prostate, the patient's age and general health, and how the patient feels about the treatment options and their side-effects. Approaches to treatment include the following.

- **'Watchful waiting'** is chosen by men who decide not to have treatment immediately if the cancer is growing slowly and not causing symptoms. Instead, they have regular check-ups so they can be closely monitored. Men who are older or have another serious illness may choose this option.
- **Surgery** usually removes the entire prostate and surrounding tissues. This operation is called a radical prostatectomy. In the past, impotence was a side-effect for nearly all men undergoing radical prostatectomy, but now doctors can usually preserve the nerves going to the penis so that men can have erections after prostate removal. Incontinence, the inability to hold urine, is common for a time after this sort of surgery. Most men regain urinary control within several weeks, but a few continue to have problems that require them to wear a device to collect urine.
- **Transurethral resection** is another kind of surgery, which cuts cancer from the prostate but does not take out the entire prostate. This operation is sometimes done to relieve symptoms caused by the tumour before other treatment, or in men who cannot have a radical prostatectomy.

- **Radiation therapy** is often used when cancer cells are found in more than one area of the body.
- **Hormone therapy** is used to suppress the male hormone, testosterone, which encourages prostate cancer cells to grow and multiply.
- **Brachytherapy** is the implantation of small seeds of radioactive iodine into the prostate using ultrasound to guide the placement of the seeds. It is quick, convenient, effective and said to cause fewer side-effects than other forms of treatment. It will be increasingly used for younger men with cancer which has not spread beyond the prostate gland.

Researchers are working on a treatment that involves injecting a genetically modified form of the virus that causes the common cold (adenovirus) into prostate cancer cells. The virus is modified so that when it enters the cancer cells it makes a chemical that transforms an inactive (pro-)drug into an active drug that stops the cancer cells multiplying and kills them. Only cancerous cells are attacked while healthy cells are unscathed. It is hoped that the combination of the GM virus and pro-drug will be used in frail men in whom surgery may be dangerous or when radiotherapy has not worked. It seems unlikely that this treatment will help your father but it may yield new hope in the future.

Breasts

Enlarged breasts

Q *I am a 38-year-old man, generally fit and well, and a non-smoker apart from the occasional dope at weekends. I have put on a bit of weight over the years, mostly as a beer gut. In the last two months, I have started to develop breasts! I am far too embarrassed to see my doctor and dread the summer when it'll be T-shirts and swimming trunks time. What could it be and what can I do about it?*

A Lots of men get enlarged breasts; sometimes it is just excess fat, but it can be due to growth of breast tissue in the same way as in women. It is called gynaecomastia when it happens to men. The phenomenon is very common at puberty, when adolescent boys who are already battling with acne and squeaky voices find to their horror that one or both breasts are enlarging. They need reassurance that, like all their other ills, it is due to hormonal fluctuations and will settle down.

Gynaecomastia is equally common in old age. The next most common cause is drugs: one example is cimetidine (Tagamet – for indigestion), and your old friend marijuana is among the culprits. Drugs are thought to increase the levels of oestrogen or prolactin, which are hormones that stimulate the growth of breast tissue. Liver disease, alcohol abuse, an overactive thyroid and testicular cancers are other rarer causes.

In extreme cases, men with gynaecomastia may need a breast reduction operation. In most cases, however, the cause is reversible and surgery is not necessary.

Breast cancer

Q *I have discovered a lump behind one of my nipples and am worried about what it might be. Can men get breast cancer?*

A It is rare, but yes, they can. Less than half a per cent of all breast cancers occur in men, it accounts for less than 1 per cent of all male cancers and is very rare indeed in men under 60 – so there is no need for men to regularly check their breasts. On average, breast cancer affects men five to ten years later than in women, so most men who develop breast cancer are over 65. The only known risk factor for male breast cancer is Klinefelter's syndrome, which is a chromosomal disorder resulting in small testicles and low male hormone levels.

Unlike gynaecomastia (see above), which causes uniform enlargement of the breast, breast cancer in men shows up as a lump under the skin or puckering of the nipple or the skin, usually to one side of the breast. Puckering of the skin and nipple is usually less noticeable in men than in women, because men have so much less breast tissue. By the time breast cancer is diagnosed in men, it is often fairly far advanced and harder to treat successfully. As in women, mammography is valuable in helping diagnosis, and a fine needle biopsy, in which a needle is put into the lump to extract cells which can be examined under a microscope, is also useful. Surgery to remove all the breast tissue, and radiotherapy, are the usual forms of treatment. Chemotherapy may be added to mop up any stray cancer cells. The drug tamoxifen (Nolvadex), which is used to treat women with breast cancer, is also given to men with the disease.

(See Chapter 5 for more about the symptoms of breast cancer.)

Male menopause

Q *Is there such a thing as the male menopause? Is there a test for it? I'm a 50-year-old man who is finding life very difficult at the moment. I seem to lack motivation, sex drive or enthusiasm for anything at work or at home. How can I find out more?*

A If we are to be precise, obviously there is no such thing as a male menopause because the word means the cessation of periods and you cannot cease what you never started. However, there is no doubt that as men get older, muscle turns to fat, and testosterone – the hormone that drives virility – becomes less rampant. This has been called 'andropause', and some experts have advocated treatment with androgen (male hormone) replacements. A blood test to check testosterone does not usually provide useful information because you can have normal levels of the hormone in your blood but become less responsive to its effects. Failing responsiveness to testosterone is a gradual process and affects everyone differently and unpredictably. The loss of enjoyment in life that you are experiencing is more likely to be due to depression than hormonal changes, and you may feel you would like to explore this further with a sympathetic partner, friend or health professional. (See Chapter 2 for more about depression.)

Chapter 5

The female body

There are very few women who have never had a gynaecological problem. Some may put up with the distress caused by severe period pains or heavy, flooding periods, although often treatment to bring relief is available. Bleeding between periods, pelvic pain or even absent periods can be very worrying. Conditions such as itching in the vulva, lumps in the groin or unpleasant vaginal discharges are not uncommon, but many women do find them embarrassing.

Solving such problems really is just part of your GP's job – but it is quite normal to feel reluctant to visit the doctor in these circumstances. You may be uncomfortable about the prospect of being examined 'down below', but this should not put you off. You can try to ensure that the person who will examine you is approachable and female, if you prefer, and you can always have a chaperone in the room to make you feel more supported. The room should be warm, comfortable and private, and any instruments used should be warmed first. Before you consent to any examination or tests you should always feel assured that you have been fully informed of why they are necessary and what is involved. If you are not comfortable with any procedure, say so. If you are not happy with your present doctor, it is not difficult to change to one with whom you feel more at ease, and you do not have to give a reason.

In addition to the gynaecological worries mentioned above, this chapter looks at genital prolapse and hysterectomy, and includes information about cervical cancer and smear tests. Premenstrual syndrome is covered in Chapter 2.

Urinary problems are much more common in women than men. Infections can happen because the female urethra is short and bacteria can travel up into the bladder easily. A surprisingly high proportion of women suffer from incontinence, which often occurs

Glossary

Amenorrhoea   Absent periods

Cervical smear test   Screening to check for abnormal cells on the cervix which are pre-cancerous

Cervix   Neck of the womb, which sits at the top of the vagina

Cystoscopy   Examination of the bladder using a 'telescope'

Dysmenorrhoea   Painful periods

Ectopic pregnancy   Fertilised egg attaches somewhere other than the uterus, most commonly in the Fallopian tube

Endometrium   Lining of the uterus

Endometriosis   A condition where the lining of the womb grows on other organs, such as the ovaries

Fallopian tube   Tube leading from each ovary to the uterus

Gynaecologist   Specialist in female reproductive problems

Hysteroscopy   Examination of the uterus using a hysteroscope (telescope), usually under general anaesthetic

Incontinence   Involuntary loss of urine

Intermenstrual bleeding   Bleeding between periods

Labia   Vaginal 'lips'

Laparoscopy   Examination of the abdominal cavity using a laparo-scope (telescope), which is inserted through the abdominal wall while you are under general anaesthetic

Menarche   Start of periods; a girl's first period

Menopause   End of periods

Menorrhagia   Heavy periods

Perineum   Skin between the vagina and the anus

Uterus   Womb

Urethra   Tube between the bladder and its opening, just in front of the vagina

Vagina   The birth canal extending from the uterus to outside the body

Vulva   Area around the vagina comprising the labia and clitoris

after childbirth, for example, when the pelvic floor muscles are weakened from too much pushing. Advice is offered here about dealing with these conditions, as well as with frequent urination and urinating during sex.

Breasts, too, cause much concern and embarrassment to many women. With the relatively high incidence of breast cancer in the West, the discovery of a lump can trigger panic and profound fear. This chapter gives advice about common causes of breast swelling, pain and lumps, as well as information about breast screening and self-examination. Nipple problems are also covered. For details of breast cosmetic surgery, see Chapter 1.

Vagina and vulval area

Common causes of vaginal and vulval discharge

Thrush Symptoms: white/yellow discharge; itchy, sore vulva (see below)

Bacterial vaginosis (BV) Symptoms: smelly, yellow-green discharge; not itchy or sore (see below and Chapter 8)

Trichomonas Symptoms: smelly, yellow/green, frothy discharge; sore (see Chapters 3 and 8)

Chlamydia Discharge may be yellow/green; cervix sore, or no symptoms (see Chapter 3)

Possible causes of vulval lumps

Herpes Symptoms: small blisters on the vulva; generally unwell (see Chapter 3 and page 134)

Warts Small lumps caused by a viral infection (see Chapter 3)

Cysts Fluid-filled lumps, which can appear in any part of the body where fluids are formed. If a cyst is squeezed, bacteria can enter it and cause infection, and it then becomes more swollen and painful

---

Vaginal discharge

Q *My GP has told me that I have thrush. I am confused as to how I could have caught it, and wonder whether you can tell me more about it?*

A You don't catch thrush from other people – it is a yeast called *Candida albicans*, which is a type of fungus that lives in your guts and exists in a delicate balance with other normal bacteria there. Anything that disturbs this balance can allow the thrush to run riot and cause irritation in the vagina.

If you have recently taken a course of antibiotics, this could have precipitated it. Antibiotics destroy harmful bacteria, which is why you take them, but they also knock out the 'good' bacteria and so upset the natural balance. Hormonal changes can also affect the acidity of the vagina, which makes thrush more likely to become a problem. This can occur if you take the contraceptive pill or get pregnant.

Thrush is the most common cause of an itchy vaginal discharge. It accounts for 30 per cent of all vaginal infections. It is not necessarily sexually transmitted, although your sexual partner may pick it up from you and then re-infect you. Thrush causes a thick, curdy, white discharge, intense vaginal itching and red and swollen-looking labia, and can also cause itchiness around the anus (back passage). Sometimes the thrush improves on its own, especially if it has been caused by antibiotics which you then stop taking.

Eating yoghurt can help by replacing 'good' bacteria, called lacto-bacillus (e.g. acidophilus), in the gut. Keeping your vagina cool with cotton knickers and avoiding synthetic tight trousers or leggings can also help the itching. Anti-fungal treatment can be bought over the counter, including clotrimazole (Canesten) cream or, better still, a pessary which you insert into your vagina. The oral tablet fluconazole (Diflucan) can be taken as a one-off treatment. It is available over the counter but is cheaper on prescription. Another prescription-only oral treatment is itraconazole (Sporanox), which can be effective if other treatments have failed.

Q *I have developed a smelly vaginal discharge which is slightly stronger after sex. This has only recently appeared and despite frequent washing it is not going away. What is it? Could it be anything infectious?*

A It sounds as though you may have bacterial vaginosis (BV), which typically causes a fishy smell after intercourse. BV is the second most common cause of vaginal discharge, after thrush. It is not sexually transmitted, although some authorities would recommend that your partner be treated also. You can have it diagnosed by asking for a high vaginal swab, in which the doctor or nurse uses a cotton-wool-tipped stick to mop up some of the discharge from the top of the vagina. The swabs are sent to a lab and results usually take a week.

The treatment for BV is a course of the antibiotic metronidazole (Flagyl), taken twice a day for a week or so. Metronidazole often causes a metallic taste in the mouth and an unpleasant facial flushing with alcohol, so you should not drink alcohol while you are taking it. BV does not affect your fertility, is not contagious and should clear up after the treatment although it can recur. It has been implicated as a possible factor in miscarriages, so if you are planning a pregnancy it is well worth making sure you are clear of the infection first.

Sore or itchy vagina or vulva

Q *I have developed a condition where the inside and outside of my vagina have become very sore and red. There is little or no discharge and no itch. Over a period of several weeks I have been swabbed for thrush and other bacteria, and although all the swabs were clear my GP has prescribed Canesten several times. This seems to make the condition worse. I cannot think what could be causing it – I do not take bubble baths or wear tights or tight trousers; I use non-biological washing powder and wear cotton knickers. Do you have any suggestions?*

A You have either got an infection or an allergy. Certainly you are doing all the right things. A sore, red vagina with little or no discharge may be caused by a bacteria of the streptococcal family. Swabs may not always show the bacteria and you may want to try a course of penicillin by mouth, which will clear it up if that is the cause. The best place to be checked out for vaginal infections is a sexually transmitted diseases (STD) clinic; not because that is necessarily what you have got, but because they have walk-in clinics and can do all the tests on the spot. Your local hospital will probably have an STD clinic which you can phone, although you may want to talk to your GP first.

It is possible that you have an allergy, although it does sound as though you are avoiding all the common allergens, i.e. bubble bath, soaps, etc. If the symptoms coincided with starting to use condoms or the cap (diaphragm), it could be that you are allergic to rubber or the spermicide. You could try taking an antihistamine by mouth (e.g. chlorpheniramine (Piriton), which is available over the counter); if that helps, it supports the theory that the problem is due to an allergic reaction. You could be referred for allergy testing if the symptoms continue.

Q *I am an 82-year-old woman in good general health. However, I am plagued by an infernal itching around my vagina and back passage, which is keeping me awake at night and making me very uncomfortable when I sit for long periods during the day. My GP said it was probably age-related dryness and gave me some oestrogen cream, which didn't help at all. Do you have any advice?*

A Water and chemicals could be exacerbating the itch, so wash infrequently – every other day should be enough – and avoid using all toiletries and creams on the itchy area. Cut your fingernails short and wear cotton gloves in bed so you can't scratch yourself raw. An antihistamine such as chlorpheniramine (Piriton), which is available without prescription, can be taken at night to lessen the itch. Your GP should examine you properly and refer you to a gynaecologist, if necessary, to make sure there is no underlying skin problem of the vulva. A fairly common condition called lichen sclerosis causes white scarred areas on the vulva and usually improves with a strong steroid ointment such as clobetasol propionate (Dermovate).

Vulval itching may be part of a more widespread skin condition, such as eczema or psoriasis (see Chapter 9). If you are itchy all over with no apparent skin problem, you may possibly have an underlying problem, for example diabetes or anaemia (see Chapter 1), which can be diagnosed by a simple blood test.

Lumps in the groin

Q *For several months I have been suffering from a severely sore and swollen throat, swollen glands, and lumps which appear inside or outside my vagina. The lumps are reddish purple, fluid-filled and very sore but do not burst. What could they be?*

A It may have been genital herpes, which is the commonest cause of vulval pain and ulceration. It is due to the same virus that causes cold sores – the herpes simplex virus, or HSV types I and II. An attack of herpes can cause a very painful vulva, pain passing urine, small red blisters and ulcers on the labia, flu-like symptoms and a general feeling of being unwell and washed-out.

The first attack you ever have usually starts after sexual intercourse with a partner who carries the virus and passes it on without realising. A first attack does not imply that your partner has been sleeping around – he may have harboured the virus for years and never had any symptoms. You can also get genital herpes after oral sex with a partner who carries the virus. Herpes does not affect your fertility, but if you had active genital herpes at the time of delivery of a baby you would be offered a caesarean section to avoid the baby catching herpes on the way out.

Once you have had genital herpes you may get recurrent attacks, though rarely as severe as the initial attack. You can pass herpes to any sexual partner you have in the future, even if you do not have the ulcers or blisters at the time. Oral medication with anti-viral drugs can lessen the severity of the attack and may help to prevent recurrences.

It is a good idea to attend a specialist genito-urinary or sexually transmitted diseases clinic so you can discuss these issues. You can get more information from the Herpes Viruses Association.*

(See Chapter 3 for more about sexually transmitted diseases and Chapter 10 for more about cold sores.)

Q *I have got two small pea-sized lumps where my leg creases at the top, I suppose on the knicker line. Initially they looked a bit like big spots but felt more like lumps of chewing gum. There was a small head to them, which went down within a few days, although I can still feel the tiny lumps under-neath now. At first I thought they were just spots but now I am a bit worried. Could it be anything serious?*

A If they had a small head on them, that suggests they were pus-filled spots. These commonly appear after shaving or waxing around the bikini line and they may persist for a long time. It is a good idea to stop shaving or waxing for at least a month and see if the lumps disappear. If they do not go away or if at any time they are growing, become tender or increase in number, they may be small lymph nodes (glands) which come up in response to infection – for example, herpes on the genitals, or other infections (not only sexu-ally transmitted ones). Lymph nodes do not develop heads like spots and they feel like small rubbery balls under the surface of the skin. They need to be checked out to detect whether there is any underlying infection that needs treating.

Lumps in the vagina or vulva

Q *I have developed a sore lump in my vagina. I went to my GP who said that I have a Bartholin's cyst or abscess. Antibiotics have not worked and I am being referred to a gynaecologist. What is a Bartholin's cyst and is there anything I can do to get rid of it?*

Smear tests and cervical cancer

Cervical cancer is the second most common cancer in women after breast cancer, accounting for about 15 per cent of all cancers in women.

In the UK, as part of the national screening programme, a cervical smear test is offered to women between the ages of 20 and 64 (and women over 64 who have not had previous normal smears) every three years. This is to detect early, pre-cancerous changes that can be easily treated to avoid the development of cervical cancer. Having an abnormal smear does not necessarily mean that you have cancer, or that you are going to develop it in the future. Screening, and treatment before cancer develops, has led to a fall in the number of cases of cervical cancer by almost half.

The smear test samples the cells on the area of the cervix where cancer begins. A metal instrument (speculum) is inserted into the vagina and then gently opened to allow a good view of the cervix. A wooden or plastic spatula is then scraped around the cervix to obtain cells. The sample is examined in the laboratory to identify any unusual-looking cells, and the results are sent back to your GP, stating the degree of abnormality, if any.

A smear may be reported as:

- **normal:** no abnormality seen, so the test is repeated after three years, or annually if the woman has had a previous abnormality
- **inadequate:** no cells from inside the cervix seen, so an accurate assessment could not be made. The smear needs to be repeated and a brush may be needed instead of the wooden spatula more usually used
- **abnormal:** some evidence of pre-cancerous cells (see below).

A A Bartholin's cyst is a harmless growth in one of the small glands that lubricate the vagina. The cyst is a fluid-filled lump that develops when the exit to the gland becomes blocked. If infection gets into the cyst, the swelling may become hard and painful and can cause an abscess. Antibiotics by mouth are usually prescribed if the cyst is infected. Small, painless swellings can often be left alone. Large cysts that keep getting infected may need to be drained in a

A smear test may also reveal severe inflammation of the cervix, often caused by infection; in such a case the test may be repeated after six months or the patient may be referred for a colposcopy (see below).

The test may detect the presence of the wart virus or other infection; appropriate treatment and follow-ups will be arranged.

If **pre-cancerous** cells are detected, the smear is classified as 'mild' (cervical intraepithelial neoplasia 1 or CIN 1), 'moderate' (CIN 2) or 'severe' (CIN 3) depending on the level of abnormality of the cells.

If you have a 'mild' abnormality reported, the test is likely to be repeated in a few months to see if the cells are still abnormal – in some cases changes in the cervix could mean that the cells return to being normal. If you have a 'moderate' or 'severe' abnormality, and a second smear confirms this you will be sent to a hospital for a colposcopy (an examination of the cervix using a modified microscope). A small sample can be taken of any abnormal-looking areas; it will be examined under a microscope for signs of pre-cancer. You do not need a general anaesthetic and should feel fine the next day. You may have some bleeding and it is wise not to have sex for about ten days to avoid infection or soreness.

You may be offered laser treatment to prevent the development of cancer; it is advisable to take it. It is estimated that over a period of 20 years, only 40 per cent of women who have 'moderately' or 'severely' abnormal' smear tests will, if untreated, go on to have cervical cancer. The other 60 per cent will stay the same or improve.

Early cervical cancer is rarely seen on smears, because the test should pick up any abnormalities in the cells in a pre-cancerous state; clearly treatment for pre-cancer is less drastic and more effective than it is for cancer. If the cancer has not spread much, it is called microinvasive carcinoma; if it has, it is called invasive carcinoma and is more serious.

small surgical operation. It is important to see your doctor or gynaecologist to check the diagnosis and discuss the treatment options. But don't panic: you will probably be reassured and advised that no immediate treatment is needed.

Q *I have found a round little lump on my cervix. I'm petrified it's cancer. What else could it be?*

A It is far more likely to be your cervix itself than anything abnormal. Or you might have a polyp, which is a harmless growth on a stalk that comes from the cells that line the inside of the cervix. Polyps may bleed after sex or produce a lot of mucus which you would notice as a clear discharge. They can be twisted or burnt off by a gynaecologist.

To be on the safe side, ask your GP to have a look at your cervix to check, and have a smear test if it is due (see page 136).

Genital prolapse

Q *I have a constant feeling of something inside me coming down – as if my womb is about to fall out of my vagina. My GP examined me and said I have a prolapse and that he would refer me to a gynaecologist. What does it mean, and what should I expect?*

A A prolapse is when one body organ falls through another part. The most common type of genital prolapse in women is when the bladder bulges into the vagina (cystocele). Another common type is where the uterus descends down the vagina (uterine descent) and the third type is where the rectum (bowel) bulges into the vagina (rectocele). These three situations can all exist at the same time. The symptoms of a prolapse are:

- sensation of a lump coming down, pain during sex and/or backache
- dragging sensation in the pelvis, particularly by the end of the day
- stress incontinence, i.e. losing urine when you cough, sneeze, etc., and a tendency to urine infections
- straining to open the bowels and constipation
- bloodstained discharge if the prolapsed part rubs on underwear.

The factors that can lead to all types of prolapse include pregnancy, childbirth, the menopause and long-term coughing or constipation, all of which put a strain on the pelvic floor muscles.

Treatment can include:

- **ring pessary** – suitable for women who do not want an operation, are elderly and infirm, or pregnant. These rings of rubber are fitted into the vagina by a doctor or nurse and hold the womb up. They need to be changed every six months or so, depending on the type used
- **hormone replacement therapy (HRT)** – improves the pelvic floor muscles, reduces urine infections and improves vaginal soreness. However, it does not really cure the prolapse
- **surgery** – there are various surgical procedures to hitch up the uterus and/or strengthen the vaginal walls to prevent the bladder or rectum prolapsing
- **hysterectomy** – this is also sometimes advised. All these surgical operations are major and take around six weeks to recover from fully.

Periods

Painful periods

Q *I get excruciating period pain every month, which completely lays me low, making me feel quite sick and miserable and usually unable to work for one or two days. I generally end up taking to my bed with a hot water bottle. Can you suggest anything to help me cope better?*

A Period pains usually start just as the period is starting, and feel like an ache in the lower abdomen, back and legs. Pelvic congestion, which is due to a build-up of blood in the veins of the pelvis, is probably to blame, and the pain passes within a few hours or couple of days. Crampy pains – which come in spasms, may last for a couple of hours and cause nausea and even vomiting – are probably due to the squeezing shut of the blood vessels in the womb by chemicals called prostaglandins.

When periods first start (the menarche) and when they are tailing off towards the menopause, the ovaries do not produce an egg each cycle. The periods that result tend to be painful and sometimes heavy. Some women find that their periods tend to improve as they get older, especially after the birth of their first child, although around the time of the menopause they may become painful again.

Possible causes of painful periods (dysmenorrhoea)

Primary dysmenorrhoea   The most common cause of painful periods. The hormone vasopressin affects the muscle of the uterus and causes the release of chemicals called prostaglandins, which cause pain

Endometriosis   (See below)

Pelvic inflammatory disease (PID)   PID is an infection of the uterus and Fallopian tubes, which can cause fever, pain on intercourse, lower abdominal pain, vaginal discharge and vaginal bleeding – although sometimes there are no symptoms at all. Untreated PID can damage the Fallopian tubes, ovaries and uterus, including the cervix, and can result in long-term chronic pelvic pain and lingering infection. It can also cause scarring that may lead to infertility. Sexually transmitted infections, such as chlamydia, can lead to PID. It is important to seek medical advice quickly in order to get an accurate diagnosis and the correct antibiotic treatment

Intrauterine device (IUD)   An IUD, or coil, can cause heavier or more painful periods, and if this is the case you might want to consider a different method of contraception

Pelvic pain syndrome   The name given to long-standing pain in the pelvic area for which no other medical cause can be found

If your period pains are particularly severe, you should be checked for endometriosis (see below) and consider whether to take the contraceptive pill.

Strategies that you could try in order to ease the pains include:

- aerobic exercise, e.g. swimming, cycling, fast walking or jogging, around period times
- warm bath or hot water bottle while the cramps are bad
- mefenamic acid (Ponstan, available on prescription only), aspirin or ibuprofen preparations, which can block the chemicals (prostaglandins) that are partly responsible for the crampy pains
- homeopathic and herbal remedies, which are available in specialised shops – although scientific evidence of their usefulness is not available.

Other treatments are available that may be helpful for painful periods. These include:

- acupuncture and cranial osteopathy (manipulation of the skull by an osteopath). Other relaxation therapies and techniques for controlling pain can also make the pains more bearable
- stronger painkillers than those available over the counter, or hormones including the contraceptive pill. These may be advised by your doctor if suitable.

Q *I suffer from very bad period pain. My doctor says I may have endometriosis, and has referred me to a gynaecologist to be tested for it. This has got me quite worried – can you tell me what exactly endometriosis is, and what the testing and treatment for it will involve?*

A Endometriosis is a condition in which the tissue that lines the womb (endometrium) is also deposited on other organs, such as the ovaries. The endometrium outside the womb becomes pumped full of blood, in the same way that the endometrium in the womb does. This causes inflammation, cysts, and bands of tissue to get stuck together (adhesions), which can cause fertility problems because the Fallopian tubes may become blocked. Period pains may become much more severe than before the endometriosis flared up. The only way to diagnose the condition with any certainty is by laparoscopy. This involves a gynaecologist inserting a laparoscope (telescope) into the abdomen, under general anaesthetic, to have a look at the ovaries and other organs.

Drugs which cause a temporary menopause and 'switch off' the ovaries, e.g. buserelin (Suprefact) may be given, or hormone treatment, e.g. danazol (Danol), advised. By stopping the body's natural hormone cycles for a while, the inflamed tissues can recover. Endometriosis may recur after treatment, but often it does not. Surgery to release adhesions and remove the cysts caused by endometriosis is occasionally necessary, especially if the problem is interfering with fertility.

Heavy periods

> **Possible causes of heavy periods (menorrhagia)**
>
> **Dysfunctional uterine bleeding (DUB)**   Hormonal imbalance
>
> **Polyps – cervical or endometrial**   Fleshy swellings that stick out of the lining of the cervix or endometrium. They are not cancerous but may bleed
>
> **Endometriosis**   The tissue that lines the womb is deposited on other organs (see above)
>
> **Fibroids**   Non-cancerous growths in the muscle layer of the womb (see below)

Q *I get incredibly heavy periods with flooding and clots. I am 38 and have three children. I don't want any more children but would also like to avoid a hysterectomy if at all possible – my mother had one and went into an early menopause as a result, as well as taking a very long time to recover. What can I do?*

A Heavy periods are a nuisance but they are not dangerous. Ask your GP to do a blood count to make sure you are not anaemic from all the blood loss. If you need contraception, why not take the contraceptive pill if you can? If the periods are painful, mefenamic acid (Ponstan) in doses of 500mg three times a day for the first four to five days of the period will help with pain and blood loss. If pain is not a problem, you could be prescribed tranexamic acid (Cyklokapron), at a dose of 1g three times a day, for the first four days of the period. This drug reduces menstrual blood loss by nearly half. A lot of doctors still prescribe hormonal treatments with progestogens, such as norethisterone, but these do not work.

If these measures are no help, there are several other good options, including the Mirena (a coil that releases the hormone progestogen into the womb – see Chapter 6) and surgical procedures that are far less drastic than a hysterectomy. Endometrial resection, for example, is an effective and safe way of controlling heavy periods and involves an operation to remove the lining of the womb (endometrium) through a hysteroscope. The endometrium can be cut away, lasered, or destroyed using microwaves.

Q *I have very heavy periods, and have now been told by my doctor that I have a uterine fibroid. Please could you tell me whether this is serious, and what the treatments are?*

A Fibroids are non-cancerous growths in the muscle layer of the womb (myometrium). Big ones that stick out of the womb can cause pressure on surrounding organs like the bowel, and cause abdominal pain, bloating, pressure on the bladder and backache. In the rare cases when the fibroid outstrips its own blood supply and grows rapidly (e.g. in pregnancy), it can cause severe pain. Often, however, there are no symptoms – although sometimes difficulty in getting pregnant can be caused by a uterine fibroid, especially if it is very large.

Fibroids that stick into the womb may be much smaller but cause more symptoms in the way of heavy and sometimes painful periods. However, many fibroids cause no problems at all and are found during an ultrasound scan (sometimes by coincidence). They tend to shrink after the menopause. If they are causing no problems, treatment is not usually necessary.

Treatment involves an operation either to cut out the fibroid itself (myomectomy) or even a complete hysterectomy. If you do not need treatment, annual ultrasound scans to keep an eye on the fibroids may be advisable.

Absent or erratic periods

Q *My daughter started her periods at age 11. Now, after two-and-a-half years, she still has gaps of several months – even, on one occasion, six months – between them. In every other way she is fine: she eats well, is a reasonable weight for her height, has a healthy sprinkling of spots, enjoys school and leisure. However, she is concerned about it. Should she be?*

A Patchy periods are just one of the many trials of adolescence and are usually nothing to worry about. The reason they are often irregular for the first couple of years is that the hormone surge required for ovulation does not happen every month. Gradually the hormones, which are controlled by the brain and produced by the ovaries, will get into their stride and your daughter will slip into the regular periods that for most women come every 21 to 35 days. If you take her to

---

Possible causes of absent periods (amenorrhoea)

Pregnancy If there is any chance at all that you could be pregnant, it is worth doing a pregnancy test if you miss a period

Stress, weight loss, travel These factors affect the part of the brain that produces hormones that stimulate the ovaries

Menopause Although for most women in the UK the menopause starts at about age 50, for some it can be much earlier (see Chapter 6)

Polycystic ovary syndrome (PCOS) This is a condition in which there are a large number of cysts on the ovaries. PCOS may cause no problems but can lead to a hormonal imbalance resulting in increased levels of male hormones (androgens). Symptoms include irregular or absent periods, excessive hairiness (hirsutism), acne and sometimes infertility. It is more common in overweight women. Treatment options include losing excess weight, taking the contraceptive pill to tackle the hormonal imbalance, or drug treatment or surgery to stimulate the ovaries

Overactive thyroid (See Chapter 1)

Drugs that affect hormones

---

your GP, be prepared to be asked whether she could be pregnant – it is the most common cause of missed periods and obviously not unheard of in young teenagers. A blood test and ultrasound scan would establish whether there is an underlying problem such as polycystic ovary syndrome (see above), which is essentially a long-term hormonal disturbance that may require treatment in time.

Q *I am 17 and my periods still haven't started. Most of my friends started when they were about 12, and they had all started by the age of 14. I think I am otherwise normal and healthy. What should I do?*

A You are almost certainly just on the late side of normal and will start your periods any month now. At the same time, it is certainly worth going to your GP for some tests just to reassure you that all is well. These might include:

- weight measurement and assessment of whether puberty has been reached (i.e. hair in armpit and pubic area and breast development)
- blood test for hormonal levels and thyroid function, vaginal examination (though not appropriate if you are a virgin) and ultrasound scan to check your womb and ovaries
- rarely, if a congenital problem is suspected, referral to hospital for examination under anaesthetic and blood tests to check chromosomes.

Often no treatment will be necessary. In the case of a minor hormonal imbalance, periods that have never started or have stopped will often (re)start spontaneously. If your lifestyle seems to be causing, or contributing to, the problem, then changes to it can often relieve the problem.

In the long term, it is not beneficial for women to go for months or years without having periods, because it implies that their ovaries are not producing the oestrogen hormone, which is important in keeping bones strong and protecting the heart. In some cases, it may also predispose them to an increased risk of cancer of the womb (endometrial cancer). If absent periods do not start (or restart) on their own, some form of hormone replacement should be offered and you may be referred to a gynaecologist who has a special interest in amenorrhoea, for specific advice.

Bleeding between periods

Q *I have been suffering from irregular periods for a number of years, as well as bleeding during or after intercourse. I am 29 years old. I have paid numerous visits to my doctor and tried many contraceptive pills, had a hysteroscopy to look inside my womb and have been checked for sexually transmitted diseases at the hospital. I am on my second attempt at taking no contraception to see if my cycle will somehow return to normal – but nothing seems to work. Where do I go from here?*

A Vaginal bleeding between periods or after intercourse is a very common problem and is usually harmless. It is important, however, to see a doctor for any abnormal vaginal bleeding, because occasionally

Causes of vaginal intermenstrual bleeding

Common causes

Breakthrough bleeding on contraceptive pill or HRT   This is harmless. Changing to a different formulation may help

Dysfunctional uterine bleeding (DUB)   DUB, or a hormonal imbalance, is the most common cause of abnormal vaginal bleeding. However, it is important to see a doctor in order to rule out more serious conditions (see below). Hormones in the form of the contraceptive pill, HRT or progestogens can usually correct any imbalance

Cervical polyp   These are small, fleshy outgrowths from the cervix or endometrium, and may cause bleeding after intercourse. They can easily be removed by a gynaecologist

Cervical erosion   This is not actually an erosion, but the name given to a natural process whereby the delicate cells that line the inside of the cervix grow on to the outer surface of the cervix where it sits at the top of the vagina. This bleeds easily if irritated by a smear test, intercourse or tampons. It can be easily treated by cauterising with a silver nitrate-tipped stick. (See Chapter 3 for more about this)

Pelvic inflammatory disease (PID)   An infection of the uterus and Fallopian tubes, which if untreated can lead to infertility (see page 140)

Less common causes

Miscarriage or ectopic pregnancy   In both cases, the previous period should have been missed (although this might not always be obvious). If in doubt, it is best to do a pregnancy test and seek medical help

Cervical cancer   Abnormal vaginal bleeding may be a sign of cancer of the cervix. This is more common among women who have had genital warts, multiple sexual partners or who smoke. Having regular smear tests (see earlier in this chapter), from the age of 20, helps to identify early changes that may eventually lead to cancer unless treated

Endometrial cancer Abnormal vaginal bleeding, especially after the menopause, may be a sign of cancer of the endometrium. It is rare in women under 50 and is less common in women who have taken the contraceptive pill. It is more common in women who are childless, older than 50, obese or had a late menopause. Oestrogen without progestogen can cause endometrial cancer, which is why women who have not had a hysterectomy need to take progestogen with their oestrogen when taking HRT. (For more about these matters, and about post-menopausal bleeding, see Chapter 6) it can be a sign of a potentially dangerous, but treatable condition like cancer of the cervix or endometrium (see box). The doctor may be able to diagnose the problem after listening to details of the symptoms and performing an internal examination. Tests are necessary if there is any doubt.

If you have had the relevant tests and been reassured there is nothing seriously wrong, you may want to consider a Mirena coil, which releases a small amount of progestogen hormone into the womb. This will give you contraception and is likely to minimise vaginal bleeding especially after the first three months. It can stay in place for five years. (See Chapter 6 for more details.)

Delaying a period

Q *I am due to get married at a time my period is due. Is there anything I can do to delay it or bring it on, so it doesn't clash with the day?*

A The easiest way by far is to go on the oral contraceptive pill. You can start it a couple of months before your wedding. If you start it on the first or second day of your period, you will have contraceptive protection straight away. You take the pill every day for three weeks, then have a week's break in which time you have a light period. If you calculate that your wedding and honeymoon coincide with the week of your period, just run one packet into the next (assuming this can be done with your particular pill preparation) rather than having a week off the pill.

If you have had a thrombosis (blood clot in the leg or lung) which means you cannot take the pill, you can take the other hormone used in the pill (progestogen) on its own to stop the bleeding. You will need to see your GP or visit your family planning clinic to get the pill or hormonal treatment, have your blood pressure checked and discuss which method is most suitable for you.

Hysterectomy

Q *I am due to have a hysterectomy after 16 years of extreme pain and heavy bleeding, with no relief after trying lots of different drugs and treatments. I feel quite apprehensive about the operation – can you tell me how I am likely to feel afterwards, and how quickly I will recover?*

A You will be in hospital for five to ten days, depending on how fast you get on your feet and when you feel able to go home. For the first 24 hours you will feel woozy from the anaesthetic. You will probably have a catheter (a tube passed into the bladder through the urethra) in to collect your urine until you can get up to wee – usually within the first day – and a drip in your arm until you can take fluids orally – again, normally within the first one or two days. You will have special stockings on until you are mobile, to prevent blood clots in the legs. Your abdomen will be sore and because your abdominal muscle layer has been cut, it will be hard for you to raise yourself from the bed and you may need to either pull yourself up by using a rail or ask for help. Raising yourself will get easier over a few days but you will still feel sore. You will not be able to bend or lift easily for a week or two and will be advised to steer clear of household tasks such as vacuuming until it feels comfortable and painless to do so.

Most women stay off work for six to twelve weeks and do not drive for at least four weeks. Obviously it depends on your job – a heavy manual job involving filling shelves and lifting boxes would be a more daunting prospect than returning to a desk job. Most women say they do not feel like sex for about six weeks or so after the operation, but you can always try sooner if you feel up to it and it does not hurt.

Having a hysterectomy often stops your ovaries working, so if you have not already experienced the menopause you may do so in the few months after the operation. You may well want to consider HRT if you get symptoms of the menopause, such as hot flushes, and should also think about HRT to prevent osteoporosis, heart disease and Alzheimer's. (See Chapter 6 for more about the menopause and HRT.)

Hysterectomy is a major operation, which should not be agreed to without considering all other options. If you do decide to go ahead, however, try to get as fit as possible before the operation – stop smoking, lose excess weight and take regular exercise if possible, as this will enhance your chances of having a smooth and rapid recovery.

Pelvic pain

Possible causes of pelvic pain

Pelvic inflammatory disease (PID)   An infection of the uterus and Fallopian tubes – see page 140

Urinary tract infection   (See later in this chapter)

Miscarriage   The loss of a pregnancy, mostly occurring in the first 12 weeks. Miscarriage affects up to 20 per cent of all known pregnancies by 12 weeks. The most common symptom is bleeding from the vagina, although pelvic pain is also very common

Ectopic pregnancy   This occurs when the fertilised egg attaches itself outside the uterus; in the majority of cases, in Fallopian tubes. In rare cases, the egg attaches itself in one of the ovaries, the cervix or another organ within the pelvis. An ectopic pregnancy is not usually capable of surviving and in most instances an embryo is not developed. It will usually miscarry, but the majority of cases diagnosed will have to be operated on or treated with medication. Symptoms include bleeding from the vagina, abdominal pain, or fainting. An ectopic pregnancy can be life-threatening if it ruptures and causes internal bleeding

Ovarian cyst   Usually harmless with no symptoms, but can cause pelvic pain and need to be removed. (See below)

Q *I have had a dull ache in my lower abdomen for a few weeks now. It comes and goes. Sometimes it is painful to pass urine, at other times I have no particular symptoms. Sex is sometimes uncomfortable. I have had a vaginal discharge in the past although that is OK now. Should I worry?*

A The possible causes of your pain include bowel problems such as irritable bowel syndrome (see Chapter 7), pelvic inflammatory disease (see page 140), urinary tract infections (see below) and swellings such as ovarian cysts (see below). If you are pregnant, pain can herald a miscarriage or an ectopic pregnancy, and both require urgent attention.

If the symptoms are intermittent, it is worth keeping a careful diary of them so you can observe their relationship to your periods and note which symptoms occur together. Show this diary to your

GP. You should have a thorough check-up including a vaginal examination, swabs for infection, a smear test if it is needed and an ultrasound scan to look for ovarian cysts. A urine test should be taken to check for infection.

Q *Around the middle of my menstrual cycle I suffer from pain low down on my left side. It is very uncomfortable but only lasts a couple of days. I have heard that it is possible to suffer from ovulation pain. Is this true?*

A It is indeed possible to suffer from ovulation pain. Two weeks before the start of your next period, one of your ovaries releases an egg. If it is fertilised, you get pregnant. If not, you shed the lining of your womb two weeks later in a period. Many women have no pain or other signs of ovulation. But some, like you, get pain (on either side of the abdomen), mood swings or changes in their vaginal mucus for a day or two when ovulating. It can be very helpful to know when you ovulate if you are trying to get pregnant, as that is your most fertile time. Painkillers such as Ponstan (mefenamic acid – although this should be avoided if you are trying to conceive), hot water bottles and aerobic exercise can all help, although the pain is not usually severe. Severe or unusual pain should always be investigated as it may be due to bowel or ovarian problems.

Q *A friend of mine has been told she may have a cyst in one of her ovaries. How serious is this? Can it become malignant, and could it affect her ability to have children?*

A Many women have ovarian cysts, which may show up on an ultrasound scan and cause no symptoms at all. The vast majority are just small collections of fluid in the ovaries that develop as part of a normal menstrual cycle and disappear on their own within a few weeks.

Other, larger cysts are almost always benign (i.e. non-cancerous) and may be related to endometriosis (see earlier in this chapter) or due to abnormally developing cells (dermoid cysts). Many are never diagnosed unless they grow and cause pain or abdominal swelling. They can also sometimes cause pain during sex and severe pain if they suddenly twist, burst or bleed. In these cases they may need to be removed in an operation. The vast majority of cysts will never affect fertility or develop into cancer. Removing an ovarian cyst should not interfere with fertility unless both ovaries have to be removed, which would be very unusual, or if there is an underlying condition, such as severe endometriosis, which is threatening fertility.

Cancerous ovarian swellings can occur but are rare, especially in younger women. Ovarian cancer does not cause cysts but a solid lump on the ovary. The average age at which it is detected is 59 and it is rare among women under 45. It can be very difficult to detect in its early stages, because it produces only vague symptoms, such as abdominal bloating, weight loss, loss of appetite, wind, backache and so on, all of which are usually due to harmless causes. Blood tests and vaginal ultrasound scanning can help to diagnose ovarian cancer, but have not proved to be reliable enough to be used in a screening programme. Treatment of ovarian cancer depends on the stage of the disease but will usually involve surgery to remove the ovaries, womb, and Fallopian tubes, in addition to chemotherapy.

Urinary problems

Blood in urine

Q *The other day I noticed some blood in my urine, and I have also had some discomfort when I wee. I feel too worried to even go the doctor. I am 23 years old. Is it likely to be cancer?*

A It is true that blood in the urine can – rarely – be the only sign of a urinary malignancy. However, the most common cause of blood in the urine is a urinary infection. Women are very prone to urinary infections because of the short length of the urethra. Unlike the male urethra, which travels down through the penis, the female urethra is surrounded by bacteria which can quite easily work their way up into the bladder.

Drinking plenty of fluids – particularly cranberry juice – helps to soothe the bladder, but if you do have bacteria in the bladder a short course of antibiotics is best. If the bleeding does not clear up after antibiotics you will be recommended to have a cystoscopy, in which a telescope is put into the bladder to check for harmless polyps and for bladder cancer.

Bladder cancer in young women is exceedingly rare. Kidney stones can also cause blood in the urine, sometimes painlessly; but usually they also cause excruciating pain and vomiting.

Sometimes, it may appear that the blood is in the urine but it may be coming from your back passage if you have piles (see Chapter 7) or from your vagina if you are having a heavy period.

Urinary infections after the menopause

Q *I had a hysterectomy at the age of 37, six years ago, and have since gone through the menopause. Last year I contracted a severe urinary tract infection which necessitated five days in hospital. Since then I have had recurring infections every three or four weeks. I saw a urologist who did various tests including scans, although the results were all normal, and prescribed long-term low-dose antibiotics (Trimethoprim). However, I am now in a vicious circle of having three weeks or so clear, then the pain again, whenever I urinate. What can I do?*

A A lot of women get recurrent urinary infections after the menopause, and constant antibiotics are clearly not a satisfactory long-term solution. The urologist would probably want to have a look inside your bladder (cystoscopy) by now, so maybe you should have a frank chat with the consultant rather than being fobbed off by junior doctors who may not appreciate how many times you have been back. The underlying problem may well be that your vagina has become dry, sore and susceptible to infections since you went through the menopause, and these infections then travel up into your bladder. HRT in the form of oestrogen pessaries or vaginal creams often helps to break the cycle of infection. HRT is available as oral tablets or patches if you prefer, and is worth a try.

(See Chapter 6 for more about the menopause and HRT.)

Incontinence

Q *What can you do for stress incontinence, apart from pelvic floor exercises? I've been told these exercises can take months to work and I have the problem now.*

A There really is no short cut for stress incontinence, which is urine leakage due to weakened bladder supports. As you will know, urine leaks out when the pressure in the bladder increases, for example, when you cough, sneeze, laugh or exercise. Stress incontinence often starts after childbirth, particularly after long and difficult vaginal deliveries where you have had to push for a long time.

To minimise pressure rises in the bladder, you should try avoiding situations that precipitate a leakage. This includes constipation, because straining to open your bowels pushes up the pressure in your bladder. Take antihistamines if you sneeze a lot because of allergies. Do not smoke, because that increases your chances of coughing a lot, and avoid exercise that makes you leak – step aerobics and horse riding are two forms of exercise that some women find they had to give up because of leakage.

Some tips that may help are:

- always empty your bladder before exercising
- restrict your fluid intake to 1.5 litres per day (though not less, and not if you find such a restriction too uncomfortable)
- put a large tampon in your vagina before exercising. (But remove it afterwards to avoid any risk of toxic shock syndrome. This is an extremely rare but potentially serious condition, caused by a bacteria that normally lives on the skin. It is more likely to occur if you forget to change a tampon and leave it in your vagina for many hours. Signs occur during a period and include high fever, a rash in which skin peels off, vomiting and diarrhoea, and dizziness and fainting.)

You *will* benefit if you persevere with pelvic floor exercises, with or without vaginal cones to help (these are graduated weights which you put in the vagina and retain there while walking around for increasing lengths of time).

Surgery is another option, but really only one to consider if the exercises are not enough, as the procedure is a major operation which will result in up to a week in hospital and at least six weeks until you are fully fit again. Surgeons claim an 85 per cent success rate after the procedure most commonly performed in the UK, which is known as colposuspension. On the other hand, although two-thirds of women say the operation results in some improvement, a recent survey found that only 28 per cent of women were totally continent one year after surgery. It depends how bad the problem is – you may be willing to put up with a bit of leakage but unable to tolerate more.

Further help and advice is available from the Continence Foundation★ and *In*contact.★

Q *I have been recommended to have an injection of Microplastique into the neck of my bladder to alleviate my stress incontinence. I have had previous surgery and been advised against a further operation. I feel nervous about this treatment, which I associate with silicones, and I think these have been shown to have harmful effects when used as implants. Can you give any advice on this?*

A An injection of collagen, or Microplastique, round the bladder neck creates a band of tissue which prevents leakage from the bladder. The injection can be done as a day case, under a short general anaesthetic or even a local. Two years after the injection, 50 per cent of women are fine but 50 per cent are leaking again. There is no evidence that the inert material used causes any widespread problems, such as tiredness or muscle aches, which is also what many experts say about silicone breast implants.

It would be advisable to try the injection before a major operation, especially if you have been advised against surgery. Ask your GP about the new technique coming to the UK, which uses a prolene mesh to prop up the urethra. Known as tension-free vaginal tape (TVT), it has been used in Scandinavia for several years and appears to be more reliable than the injections and less invasive than an operation.

Urinating during sex

Q *Sometimes I leak urine when having sex. It is excruciatingly embarrassing. At first, my partner thought I was having a particularly good orgasm with lots of vaginal fluids. But in the morning, the sheets often smell faintly of urine and I'm certain that I am actually weeing a bit during sex. What can I do?*

A Your problem of passing some urine during sex without being unable to control it is a fairly common one, but because most women keep quiet about it and rarely discuss it with their doctor, it is hard to know how many women are affected.

Essentially, your problem is the same as urge incontinence (see 'Frequent urinating', below), in which the nerves in the bladder wall send messages to the brain to empty the bladder even when it is not really full. This is also known as detrusor instability.

A few self-help measures may do the trick:

- try not to drink too much in the two or three hours before sex. Avoid caffeine and alcohol because they act as diuretics and encourage you to produce more urine
- empty your bladder before sex
- avoid sexual positions that increase the pressure unduly. There is no one position guaranteed to do this but try to keep a mental note as to which positions make it worse
- avoid getting drunk – it makes it harder to exert mental control over your continence.

You could consider getting medication which is used in the treatment of urge incontinence (see page 156), and take a tablet an hour or so before sex rather than on a continuous basis.

If the problem remains embarrassingly frequent, starts to interfere with your enjoyment of sex or is associated with other signs of urge or stress incontinence such as wetting yourself when you run, it is time to seek professional help (see 'Incontinence', above).

Urine dark and cloudy

Q *I have noticed that at times my urine is extremely strong-smelling, cloudy and dark in colour. This has occurred since I had an extended bout of 'flu a few months ago. What is the likely cause of it?*

A The likely cause is that you are not drinking enough fluids and that your urine is concentrated. In itself, this is not dangerous, but may be a signal to you that your kidneys are having to extract all the fluid they can from the urine, leaving it dark and strong-smelling. If, for example, you rely on coffee as your sole source of fluid intake, you may well be dehydrated despite drinking several cups a day. This is because the caffeine in coffee is a diuretic, so the more you drink, the more fluid your body gets rid of. (A diuretic is a drug that acts on the kidneys to increase the amount of fluid that goes in to the urine. Diuretics are sometimes called 'water pills', but they actually do the opposite, making the body get rid of more fluid.) Try drinking an extra six glasses of water a day and cutting out coffee and cola, and see whether your urine lightens up.

It is worth asking your GP or practice nurse to check your urine for protein, which can indicate kidney disease, and to send it to the lab to check there is no infection. They can also check for glucose. Dark urine can also be a sign of jaundice, caused by a gallstone blocking the exit to the liver, for example. In that case, however, you would also have pale, clay-coloured stools, yellow whites of the eyes, and itchy skin.

Frequent urinating

Q *For about four years now I have had to go to the toilet to wee excessively often, and each time I go I usually wee a lot. In a typical day I go about 25 or 30 times, and usually two or three times at night. I have had an ultrasound scan and been tested for diabetes, but both tests showed no problems. I now feel as though my doctor no longer wants to help me as he has said there is nothing more he can do. Could it be an allergy? I feel very frustrated as this problem is really getting me down.*

A It is unlikely that allergy is a cause, but you have what is known as urge incontinence – even though you are not incontinent. Normally, when the bladder is full the bladder wall fires off a message to the brain saying that it needs emptying. In some people, however, their bladder wall becomes oversensitive and sends a message to the brain when the bladder is only a little full. The trick is to retrain your bladder. Try going to the toilet every half-hour, whether you need to or not. Then lengthen this period so eventually you go every two to three hours whether you want to or not. Try not to go between these times. Within a few weeks, you should be back to normal. You may need expert help with this retraining programme. Drugs such as oxybutynin (Ditropan) can also help, although it tends to cause a dry mouth.

Breasts

Swollen or painful breasts

Q *My breasts get very swollen and tender for the week before my period – that's a quarter of my life! My GP offered me various drugs but said they all have potential side-effects that sound even worse than the breast pain. Can you suggest anything else?*

A It may be a comfort for you to know that there is absolutely no link between the sort of pre-period breast pain and lumpiness that

Possible causes of breast pain

Premenstrual   Worse before periods

Hormonal   Owing to oestrogens: pregnancy, the contraceptive pill or HRT

Mastitis   Inflammation while breastfeeding

Bornholm's disease   A viral infection causing inflammation of the muscles between the ribs and sudden pain in the side of the chest (usually in young adults)

Tietze's syndrome   Inflammation of the ribs near where they meet the breasts; cause unknown

Heart disease   e.g. angina (See Chapter 1)

Gallstones   Stones in the gallbladder, which lies in the upper right-hand corner of the abdomen; can cause nausea and pain, and occasionally fever and jaundice

Possible causes of breast lumps

Cysts or **skin cysts (sebaceous cysts)**   Fluid-filled swellings

Fibroadenoma   Non-cancerous lump, which may move around

Mastitis and **breast abscess** while breastfeeding

Fat lumps (lipoma)

Breast cancer   (See below)

you may get, and breast cancer. And although your breasts are obviously sensitive to the hormone shifts that occur just before a period, this does not mean there is anything unusual or abnormal about your hormone levels.

You can try the following:

- wear a soft bra at night
- avoid heavy exercise and repeated lifting
- consider stopping hormones you may be taking, e.g. the contraceptive pill, mini-pill or HRT (see Chapter 6 for more about these)
- reduce fats in your diet, especially saturated fats, e.g. animal fats
- evening primrose oil – see below.

The usual dose of evening primrose oil is 6–8 (40mg) capsules a day, spread out over three doses a day. The usual preparation is Efamast, which contains 40mg of gamolenic acid in each capsule. It is taken daily for at least four months, and may cause mild nausea but no other side-effects. About 45 per cent of women who take it will be helped by it, though the improvement may take three months to become apparent. It is best to take it for six months at a time, then stop. The pain often recurs in about half of those whose symptoms have improved, but it may well be less severe. A further six-month course can help if severe pain recurs.

(See Chapter 2 for more about pre-menstrual syndrome.)

Breast lumps

Q *I am 27 and have recently discovered a lump in my breast, which is quite hard and sometimes painful. My GP has said she thinks it might be a cyst, and doesn't think it's cancer, but she is now referring me to have it seen and obviously I am worried. As far as I know I have no other female relatives with breast cancer. What is the risk that I have cancer?*

A Statistically your risk is low, as breast cancer usually affects older women or younger women with a strong family history of the disease. Cysts feel different from cancer – cysts are round with a regular outline whereas cancerous lumps tend to be fixed, hard and irregular in shape. However, in practice it is not always possible to tell the difference between a benign and a malignant lump. An ultrasound scan will be able to differentiate between a cyst and cancer in most cases. You should certainly be seen by a specialist within two weeks, as if it is cancer, the sooner you start treatment the better. If you do not have an appointment within that time, you should let your GP know.

Breast cancer

Breast cancer affects one in 12 women in the UK and is the main cause of death from cancer among women in England. Some 5 per cent of women die from breast cancer: the rest die of other causes such as heart disease, strokes, other cancers and old age. Most cases of breast cancer occur in women over 50. It is uncommon in women under 30, and the chances of getting breast cancer rise as you get older. It is very rare indeed among men. As with any cancer, the earlier breast cancer is detected, the higher the chances of survival. About 70 per cent of all women diagnosed with breast cancer are still alive five years later, and many die of an unrelated disease.

The aim of screening is to detect breast cancer while it is still in its early stages and before it has a chance to spread. Breast examination either by yourself or by a health professional may not be an effective way of screening for breast cancer, although most women feel that checking for breast lumps at regular intervals is helpful.

No one knows what causes breast cancer. It is more common in developed countries and appears to be related to lifestyle and possibly the amount of fat in the diet. Educated women who live in affluent Western cities are most at risk. Fewer than one in five cases of breast cancer is thought to be due to an inherited tendency. But a woman who has a sister, mother or daughter with breast cancer may be more prone to the disease. Having had breast cancer in the past increases your risk of developing another lump, and some kinds of non-cancerous breast lumps may predispose you to developing breast cancer. Women who have their first baby over the age of 35 are at greater risk than those who became mothers for the first time before the age of 20. It is not yet clear whether the oral contraceptive pill and HRT increase the risk of breast cancer: researchers have produced contradictory conclusions.

Breast cancer usually causes a lump which is painless, or a bloodstained discharge from the nipple. Investigations include ultrasound scan, mammography (an X-ray of the breasts) and sampling of the lump (fine needle aspiration, FNA). Treatment of breast cancer involves an operation to remove the lump (lumpectomy) or removal of the whole breast (mastectomy), followed by radiotherapy or chemotherapy to prevent the spread of the disease.

Breast awareness

Breast awareness is the greatest defence there is against breast cancer. Early detection of the disease can significantly increase the chances of successful treatment.

Being breast aware means knowing how your breasts look and feel and being able to notice any unusual changes. Knowing your breasts' usual appearance can make all the difference. Men, too, need to be aware of any changes in their breast tissue, as approximately 200 men in the UK get breast cancer each year.

The appearance of your breasts will vary throughout life, as you experience menstruation, pregnancy, breast-feeding, weight loss/gain and menopause.

The best way is to check your breasts at a set time each month, for example, after a period. You need to be aware of any abnormal or unusual changes in appearance, at which point you should contact your GP immediately.

The following is a five-point plan for checking your breasts.

1. Know what is normal for you
2. Know what changes to look for
3. Look and feel
4. Report any changes without delay
5. Go for breast screening if aged 50 or over.

This is what you should look and feel for:

- any unusual change in the shape or size of one of your breasts
- whether one breast has changed and become lower than the other
- a change in the colour of the skin or a rash
- puckering or dimpling of the skin
- a nipple which has become pulled in or changed its position or shape
- any swellings under either armpit or around the collarbone (where the lymph nodes or glands are)
- discharge from one or both nipples
- constant pain in one part of your breasts or in your armpit.

Nipples

Q *My mother-in-law has told me that she recently had a clear discharge from one of her nipples that had a bit of blood in it. She is 73. She can't feel a lump. Is it something to worry about?*

A Emphatically, yes. Without wanting to alarm her, discharge from one nipple can be a sign of a blocked milk duct, a harmless growth (see above) or an underlying cancer. She needs urgent referral to a specialist breast unit by her GP. They will do a mammogram and see whether she needs further tests.

Q *In the last week my nipples have been extremely sore, weeping and itchy. I can't feel any lumps in my breasts but I am very worried about it. I am 24. Can you advise?*

A There are two likely causes. If you have started running or jogging recently, your nipples may be rubbing against your top and becoming irritated by the friction. A well-padded sports bra and Vaseline on the nipples will sort that out. The other possibility is that you have changed your soap powder and that soap residues in your clothes are irritating the skin of your nipples. Washing your clothes in a non-biological, hypoallergenic powder should prevent a recurrence, and 1 per cent hydrocortisone cream on the nipples will soothe the irritation. If it does not clear up within a week you should see your GP.

Q *I have had hair around my nipples for quite a few years. Is there any way I can get rid of it? I have heard that it is something to do with a hormonal imbalance.*

A You do not necessarily have a hormonal imbalance. Lots of women have hair around their nipples: it is particularly common among women from Mediterranean countries and for those with dark hair. It also tends to run in families. If your periods are regular, you are not likely to have a hormonal imbalance. If you have very irregular periods and other hormone-related problems, such as acne, you may want to have some blood tests and an ultrasound of your ovaries to check for conditions such as polycystic ovary syndrome (see page 144), which can cause excessive hair growth, irregular periods and acne.

It is quite probable that all the tests will be normal. The best option is to learn to live with it, especially if your partner is not bothered by it.

Ways of disguising or removing the hair include bleaching, waxing, depilatory (hair-removing) creams, plucking, electrolysis or laser treatment. None guarantees that the hair will not regrow, and all can be uncomfortable. One type of contraceptive pill, Dianette, which contains an anti-male-hormone component, is useful in controlling excess hair growth and may help to control the hair around your nipples.

(See Chapter 9 for more about unwanted hair.)

Q *I have recently noticed small spots or bumps encircling both my nipples, and the sides of my breasts also feel quite tender. I have made an appointment with my doctor, but wondered if you could tell me whether it is likely to be anything serious?*

A All women have small openings, for the milk ducts, around the nipple in the brown area known as the areola. The openings may look more prominent when you are pregnant, while breastfeeding or if your breasts change shape. For instance, if you put on weight or start the pill your breasts may get bigger and you may become more aware of the way your areola looks.

If your breasts have become tender recently, you could well have focused on them more than usual and noticed the small openings for the first time, although they may have been there all along.

It is obviously sensible to get your breasts checked and to check your own breasts for lumps (see above). It is unlikely that the small bumps you describe are anything at all to worry about.

Q *My nipples don't poke out like many women's do and I am worried that I will never be able to breastfeed and that they look unattractive. Is there anything I can do?*

A Nipples, like breasts, come in all shapes and sizes and there is no such thing as normal, better or worse ones. Nipples that have always been inverted (pointing in rather than out) are not a problem at all – that is just the way you are made. But if one of your nipples suddenly changes from a nipple that sticks out to one that is pulled in, you must seek urgent medical advice because it can signify an underlying lump.

You may well be able to breastfeed without any problem and even if your nipples are very inverted, you can always use breast-shields to help the baby to suck.

Chapter 6

Contraception, fertility and the menopause

Issues relating to fertility (whether we want to conceive or want to make sure we don't) may be hard to discuss with health professionals because they concern a very private area of our lives – the hopes and risks associated with our most intimate relationships. We may be reluctant to 'medicalise' our lovemaking – but with such potentially life-changing consequences, it is important to make an informed decision about the options that are available.

This chapter offers a realistic assessment of the pros and cons of the available methods of contraception, including sterilisation; helping you to make the best choice for your needs and circumstances. Advice about emergency contraception and abortion is included. It also looks at common causes of infertility and possible methods of assisted conception. It discusses the issue of living with childlessness, and provides details of relevant support organisations.

The menopause is a natural process that for some women presents embarrassing and uncomfortable symptoms, often severely disrupting their lives. Hot flushes can be humiliating and debilitating, mood swings can put a strain on relationships, and a dry, sore vagina may make sex painful or impossible. Many women who are going through the menopause face the crucial decision of whether to take HRT to gain relief from these symptoms and effects. The merits of HRT in its various forms are presented here, alongside the health concerns relating to it, and a discussion of natural alternatives.

> ## Glossary
>
> **Cervix**   Neck of the womb, which sits at the top of the vagina
>
> **Ectopic pregnancy**   Fertilised egg attaches somewhere other than the uterus, most commonly in the Fallopian tube
>
> **Endometrium**   Lining of the uterus
>
> **Fallopian tube**   Tube leading from each ovary to the uterus
>
> **Hormone replacement therapy (HRT)**   Hormones prescribed after the menopause to replace the oestrogen, which is no longer produced by the ovaries
>
> **Hysteroscopy**   Examination of the uterus using a hysteroscope (telescope), which is put up the vagina and into the uterus, usually under general anaesthetic
>
> **Laparoscopy**   Examination of the abdominal cavity using a laparoscope (telescope), which is inserted through the abdominal wall while you are under general anaesthetic
>
> **Ovary**   Organ on each side of the abdomen containing eggs, also producing hormones (oestrogen and progesterone)
>
> **Ovulate**   Release of an egg from the ovary
>
> **Uterus**   Womb

Contraception

In spite of the wide range of contraceptive methods available today, with more on the horizon, there is no such thing as fail-safe contraception with no side-effects. They also vary in the degree of protection they offer against sexually transmitted infections. Hormonal methods, which are some of the most reliable at preventing pregnancy, also present certain health concerns. Barrier methods are less reliable, but more effective at protecting against sexually transmitted diseases. Which you choose will depend on what is most important for you at your present stage of life.

Which contraceptive method?

Q *My 16-year-old daughter has started having sex with her boyfriend, which, I must say, I'm not too happy about. Of course I want to make sure* *she doesn't get pregnant – could you suggest what the best contraception would be for her, and how to broach the subject?*

A Good for you for facing up to the facts rather than pretending it is not happening. Your daughter probably knows a lot about sexual health and contraception, as do most young people today, but it is safest not to assume that she has been to a family planning clinic or a GP to discuss the options – or that she has acted on the advice.

Condoms are good because they help to protect against sexually transmitted diseases (STDs), but they do not offer the same level of protection against pregnancy as the combined contraceptive pill. You would probably prefer your daughter to take a belt-and-braces approach – that is, condoms to protect against STDs and the pill to protect against pregnancy. She should also know about the availability of emergency contraception over the counter (and the £25 that it currently costs). This may sound like overkill but this approach is preferable to an unwanted pregnancy, having to go through a termination, or catching an STD that may impair her fertility in the future.

As to how to broach the subject, it may be advisable to separate the discussion about these practical aspects of family planning from any debate about whether sleeping with a boyfriend at 16 is what she really wants or needs to do.

Q *I have recently embarked on my first sexual relationship and need a clear idea of the options that are available for contraception. Could you explain what each of the different methods are and which might be the safest and most reliable?*

A There really is no such thing as the ideal contraceptive – each has its pros and cons, which are briefly summarised below.

You can buy male condoms from vending machines almost anywhere. Pharmacists sell female and male condoms, emergency contraception and kits to aid fertility awareness. The combined pill, mini-pill, caps, coils, condoms, contraceptive implants and injections are all available from NHS and private family planning clinics, and GPs' surgeries.

The various methods available are as follows.

- **Combined oral contraceptive pill** This contains two hormones which are similar to the two naturally-occurring hormones produced by the ovaries, oestrogen and progesterone. The hormones in the pill override the normal hormonal cycle and so prevent ovulation, and it is very effective as long as it is taken regularly. One disadvantage is a slightly increased risk of thrombosis (blood clots in the legs or lungs). This risk is much higher among smokers. Certain side-effects, such as intermittent vaginal bleeding, headaches, acne and weight gain, are also common (see below).

- **Progesterone-only pill (mini-pill)** As this pill does not contain oestrogen, it is safe for women who, because of an increased risk of thrombosis, are unable to take the combined contraceptive pill. However, it is less reliable than the combined pill, and the pills must be taken within the same three-hour period every day to be fully effective. The mini-pill works by changing the mucus in the cervix so that sperm cannot get through, and the lining of the womb so that implantation of an egg cannot occur. Possible side-effects include acne, headaches and bloating, and it can also cause breakthrough bleeding and ovarian cysts (see Chapter 5).

- **Injectable contraceptive (e.g. Depo-provera)** This is an injection of a hormone similar to progesterone every 12 weeks. It is very effective, and periods may stop altogether. Possible side-effects include breakthrough bleeding and sometimes changes in weight or blood pressure. A disadvantage is that once you have an injection, you have to live with any side-effects for three months until it wears off.

- **Implants** As with injections, other long-acting forms of progestogen can be implanted under the skin of the arm. These last for three to five years and must be inserted and removed by a specially trained doctor. The insertion and removal can cause bruising. Irregular bleeding, as well as other side-effects, may occur for the first six months.

- **Condoms** The male condom is a rubber sheath with a teat at the end. It is rolled on to the erect penis and removed after intercourse. It does not require special fitting, and provides protection against STDs, including HIV. (See Chapter 3 for more about STDs, condom use and safe sex practices.) However, it is not as reliable as, for example, hormonal methods of contraception, as it can split or come off, and it can also interfere with the spontaneity and enjoyment of sex. The female condom is a soft sheath which is put inside the vagina before sex and removed afterwards. It offers similar protection to the male version, with the drawbacks that it can be fiddly to use, and the penis can slip in between the sheath and the vaginal wall. Some women find they are unable to retain one in their vagina. Both male and female condoms can sometimes cause allergies.

- **Diaphragm (cap)** This is a rubber dome, fitted to individual size, which fits over the cervix. It is inserted into the vagina before sex, with spermicide (sperm-killing) gel to increase its effectiveness, and left in place for six hours afterwards. Unlike the pill, the cap protects against STDs, including HIV, and it does not cause widespread changes within the body. However, it can be messy, can sometimes cause irritation or allergies, and can make sex less spontaneous, as you have to remember to insert the cap beforehand.

- **Intrauterine device (IUD) or 'coil'** This is a small copper and plastic device which is inserted into the womb by a doctor, and prevents a fertilised egg from implanting. It can remain in place for three to five years, with annual checks. Disadvantages are that it can be painful when inserted and it often causes heavier and more painful periods. If you get a sexually transmitted infection, it may spread faster with the coil and if you get pregnant with a coil, it is more likely that the pregnancy will be ectopic (see Chapter 5).

- **Levonorgestrel-containing IUD (Mirena)** This is a coil that releases small amounts of progestogen hormone into the womb, and has all the advantages of a normal coil without the heavy or painful periods. It is also used for women with heavy periods even if they do not require contraception. It is wider than the normal coil, and so insertion can be painful or require a local anaesthetic. It can cause intermittent bleeding and, like the mini-pill, some side-effects.

- **Sterilisation** The most effective form of contraception. As it is nearly always irreversible, however, you have to be very certain that you do not want any more children before deciding to opt for it. In men, the tube that takes sperm from the testicles is cut; in women the Fallopian tubes are tied or cut. Reversing male or female sterilisation is sometimes attempted but is usually unsuccessful.

- **Natural family planning (NFP)** Also known as fertility awareness, this method involves abstaining from sex at the times when the woman is fertile. It relies on her careful observation of the changes that occur during her monthly cycle, such as in body temperature and vaginal mucus. It particularly suits couples with religious or moral objections to artificial contraception, and is more reliable than no contraception, but less reliable than other methods. More information about NFP is available from Fertility UK.★

The order of effectiveness of these contraceptive methods is as follows: male sterilisation (vasectomy), female sterilisation, injectable and implantable progestogens, combined oral contraceptive pill, progestogen-only pill, coils, diaphragm, condoms, spermicides, natural family planning.

There is, however, some overlap. For example, a careful cap user may have better protection than a haphazard pill taker!

The pill

Breakthough bleeding

Q *I started taking the pill several months ago. Now I have suddenly started to bleed – in the middle of the three pill weeks, not during the week off. What does this mean? Could it be anything serious?*

A Bleeding while you are on the pill can be worrying, but it is usually due to inadequate levels of hormones in the pill for you. This may come about because:

- you have missed a few pills
- you have had diarrhoea or vomiting, so have not absorbed the pill from your gut
- you are taking other medication that interferes with the pill, e.g. drugs against epilepsy
- the hormones in the pill are not at high enough levels for you.

Other possible reasons are:

- you are pregnant and bleeding is due to miscarriage
- the bleeding is due to an infection, a 'cervical erosion' (raw patch on your cervix) or polyp (see Chapter 5 for more about these).

If you have missed pills, had diarrhoea or vomiting, or think there might be an interaction with other medication you are on, you should discuss the situation with your doctor. You might be advised to use extra contraception or change to a different pill. If the bleeding has no obvious cause, you should have a smear test and appropriate examinations to make sure there is no other underlying cause, such as an infection.

If you have any concern that you may be pregnant, it is worth doing a pregnancy test. If you are pregnant, the pregnancy test should show positive even though you are on the pill. (And if you *are* pregnant, you should stop taking the pill.) If it is negative, you can repeat the test two weeks later.

Once you have eliminated all these possibilities, then you need a pill that is relatively high in the hormone progestogen. This is similar to the naturally occurring hormone, progesterone, which keeps the lining of the womb in place. Loestrin 30 is a high-progestogen type worth trying. Alternatively, one of the triphasic pills, such as Trinordiol, may be good because they mimic your own natural cycle more closely than those pills which deliver the same strength of hormones throughout the month.

Risks and side-effects

Q *I have been on the pill for six years now, and would love to carry on with it, because it suits me fine and gives me no trouble. However, I am worried about the safety. Is it definitely safe?*

A It is a question of balancing the known benefits of the combined pill against the risks. For most women, the risk of getting pregnant is more serious than the risks associated with taking the pill, and the pill also confers some health benefits that counter the risks. Over the years the pill has often been blamed for side-effects which were in fact due to other causes.

The positive effects are that it protects against cancer of the ovary, cancer of the uterus and pelvic inflammatory disease (PID), and reduces the risk of fibroids (non-cancerous swellings in the uterus), ovarian cysts and non-cancerous breast disease (see Chapter 5 for more about all these).

On the negative side, you may get side-effects on the pill. These include nausea, breast tenderness, bleeding between periods, weight gain, headaches and mood swings. These side-effects should stop within about three months. If they do not, changing your type of pill may help. The pill may also sometimes cause an increase in blood pressure.

There are some known serious side-effects, but these are rare. A very small number of women may develop a thrombosis (blood clot), which can block a vein in the calf (deep vein thrombosis), lung (pulmonary embolus), heart (heart attack) or brain (stroke). That is why if you have ever had any of these conditions, you cannot take the pill. If there is a history of thrombosis in your family, you must seek expert help before taking the pill because tests can be done to see whether you are at increased risk yourself.

The risk of thrombosis is greatest if any of the following apply to you: you are overweight, are immobile (use a wheelchair), or a member of your immediate family had a venous thrombosis before they were 45. If you smoke, are diabetic, have high blood pressure, or a member of your immediate family had a heart attack or stroke before they were 45, you should also steer clear of the pill.

The older type of pills, such as Microgynon, has a slightly lower risk of causing thrombosis than newer pills such as Marvelon. But many women who are at low risk of thrombosis are prepared to take that small extra risk because the newer pills tend to cause fewer side-effects such as breast tenderness.

It seems that taking the contraceptive pill may slightly increase the risk of being diagnosed with breast cancer although some studies have suggested no heightened risk. If a woman stops taking the pill, within ten years any small increased risk reverts to the same as that of a woman who has never taken the pill. There is a possible increased risk of cervical cancer among pill-takers and a higher chance of developing a very rare form of liver cancer. Overall, those who take the pill do not die younger than those who do not.

Women who should not take the combined oral contraceptive pill

You should not take the combined pill if you have now or have had in the past:

- thrombosis or close family members with thrombosis
- risk factors for venous thrombosis (e.g. you are immobile)
- more than one risk factor for heart disease (e.g. you are a smoker and have high cholesterol)
- diabetes with damage to blood vessels
- uncontrolled high blood pressure
- severe liver diseases
- breast cancer or any other cancer dependent on hormones
- undiagnosed vaginal bleeding
- some types of migraine (see below).

Q *I have been taking the pill for many years, but recently I have been getting migraines more often than usual, and am concerned that this is due to the pill. Should I stop taking it?*

A Most migraine sufferers can actually safely take the combined pill, although doctors often give conflicting advice. The women who must avoid the combined pill are those who get migraine with an aura. This unpleasant and fairly rare phenomenon causes visual disturbances – such as loss of half of the visual field or zig-zag shapes that move across your visual field and seem to grow – just before the headache starts. (See Chapter 10 for more about migraine.) The worry is that women who get migraine with an aura may be more at risk of strokes and that taking the pill will increase that risk even further.

The other groups of women who are at increased risk of having a stroke while on the combined pill are heavy smokers, obese women and those with a family history of strokes and heart attacks under the age of 45. You may feel that even without an increased risk of stroke, you would rather try a different method of contraception. Your options would include the mini-pill (progestogen only), or a cap or coil if you want a non-hormonal alternative.

For further advice, contact the Migraine Action Association.*

Condoms

Q *I would really prefer my boyfriend to use condoms, but he says they often burst when he uses them and that he can't feel much when he wears one. Can you give any advice?*

A Up to 5 per cent of condoms do burst, even among experienced users, which is why they are not the most reliable method of contraception. If it is very important to you that you do not get pregnant, it would be advisable to use a different method (see earlier in this chapter). You can use condoms as well if you want to ensure protection against sexually transmitted infections.

If a condom bursts once, you can chalk it up to experience. If it keeps happening, however, check that you are pinching out the air at the top and that you are not catching the condom on sharp rings, fingernails or other objects. It may be a good idea to use extra-strong condoms with additional lubricants. Condoms that are made from polyurethane, rather than latex, are available, and are particularly good if you are allergic to latex, as 1 per cent of people are. These condoms can hardly be felt, seen or smelt, so are popular with men who do not like using condoms because of the decreased sensation and enjoyment. They are, however, expensive.

Sterilisation

Q *I recently became pregnant and had to undergo a termination, as neither my partner nor I wants children. The whole experience was extremely distressing and we want to make quite sure that it doesn't happen again, and are therefore seriously considering sterilisation for one of us. Could you tell me something about what we should know before making a decision?*

A Sterilisation is an increasingly popular method of contraception, which 45 per cent of couples in their forties, in England and Wales, opt for. Both male sterilisation (vasectomy) and female sterilisation are available on the NHS (referral via your GP) and are also offered by private clinics. Both male and female sterilisation should be regarded as being irreversible. An operation to reverse it can be attempted, but is generally unsuccessful.

Female sterilisation can be done under a local anaesthetic, although a general is preferred by the vast majority of women. A laparoscope (telescope) is introduced into the abdomen via two small incisions in the abdominal wall. The Fallopian tubes (leading from the ovaries to the womb) are tied, cut or clipped to stop any eggs released from the ovaries being fertilised. There may be some discomfort after the operation but there should be no long-term problems or need for further attention. Periods do not change after female sterilisation and it provides very good contraception, with only four pregnancies per 1,000 sterilised women per year. In the highly unlikely event of pregnancy, an ectopic pregnancy is more likely, but overall it is a very low risk indeed.

The operation for male sterilisation (vasectomy) is just as effective as female sterilisation. It is done under local anaesthetic, and involves making a cut in the scrotum and cutting or burning the 'vas deferens' – the tube that takes sperm from the testicles to the penis. It does not affect sexual performance or masculinity in any way, but there may be some discomfort and bruising of the scrotum after the operation. Occasionally female partners of men who have had a vasectomy notice that their periods are heavier.

Repeat sperm counts (two or three) are required after a vasectomy before a man can be reassured that he will not get his partner pregnant. Until then, couples need to use other contraception.

Before sterilisation, you will speak to a counsellor, often a trained nurse, who will explain everything you need to know before making a decision.

Emergency contraception

Q *I have had to use emergency contraception twice in the past six months when condoms have split. I am a bit worried about the possible effects of it on my health. Can you tell me if there are any dangers, or whether it could affect my ability to have children in the future?*

A There are three methods of emergency (postcoital) contraception currently available. Two of these are hormonal and must be taken within 72 hours of unprotected intercourse (Schering PC4 contains oestrogen and progestogen, whereas the Levonelle-2, which is now on sale over the counter, contains progestogen alone). The other method is to have a coil (intrauterine device or IUD) fitted within five days of unprotected intercourse.

Virtually any woman can take emergency contraceptive pills as long as she has not already established that she is pregnant. If you need to take them again as a one-off, that should be fine. There are no known long-term health risks associated with using postcoital contraception several times. However, it is not ideal: the doses of hormones that you are taking are high and can make you feel sick, the prescription may be difficult to obtain (e.g. at weekends), and if you buy it over the counter it is expensive. If you have a coil fitted as emergency contraception, it can then be left in your womb for up to five years and will provide good contraception for that time. But if you find you are needing to rush out to buy the emergency pill on more than one occasion, it is definitely a good idea to go to a family planning clinic or your GP for more appropriate contraception.

Abortion

Q *I have just discovered that I am pregnant but I am in no position to have a baby at this stage of my life. I want to have an abortion. Can you tell me whether I can take the abortion pill and how I should go about it?*

A The abortion pill (as opposed to postcoital contraception) is not readily available at NHS centres, and most women would not be offered it. You can get a termination of your pregnancy (abortion) on the NHS via your GP or a family planning clinic, or you can approach a private agency such as the British Pregnancy Advisory Service.★

Before you go in for a termination you should think through the issues carefully. Having a termination may be a minor procedure physically, but it could have a bigger impact on you psychologically than you imagine. You could talk through your feelings with your partner, or a friend whose opinion you value, or a professional counsellor.

There are two ways in which a pregnancy can be terminated: surgical and medical. In a surgical termination (which is used only in the first three months of the pregnancy), you are likely to have a short operation under a general anaesthetic. An instrument is inserted up your vagina and into your womb and the contents are sucked out. This is known as suction termination. When you wake up, you may have the same amount of pain and bleeding as you do when you have a period. You may feel woozy from the anaesthetic for a day or two but will be able to return to work usually within a couple of days. The psychological impact may last longer especially if you were ambivalent about having a termination in the first place (see below for advice on counselling).

A medical termination of pregnancy induces a miscarriage using drugs that block the hormone progesterone so that the pregnancy cannot continue. You will be given some pills to take, and two days later you will be given a pessary that you insert in your vagina to start the womb contracting. In about 90 per cent of cases, the pregnancy terminates fully within 12 hours of the second dose and the womb empties itself. If the termination is incomplete and tissue remains in the womb (see below for symptoms), a surgical emptying of the womb will be necessary.

Your body returns to normal rapidly after a termination though it may take some days for hormonal levels to fall and you may experience mood swings and feel tearful and vulnerable. Vaginal bleeding and abdominal cramps settle after a few days. Your first period may come a month later or may be slightly delayed. You can be fertile at any time after a termination so it is wise to use contraception from immediately after a termination. Excessive pain, bleeding or a smelly vaginal discharge may all be signs of an infection resulting from the termination, or mean that the termination was incomplete and tissue remains inside you. See a doctor if these uncommon complications occur.

A termination should not affect your fertility or damage you health in any way. Complications after a surgical termination are usually relatively minor (e.g. bleeding or an infection); major ones such as puncturing of the womb are very rare indeed.

It is common to feel psychologically battered after a termination. You may be convinced that you have done the responsible and rational thing, but still feel some regret for the baby that might have been. It is quite normal to feel that way and it is good to acknowledge and share your feelings with someone you trust. Your feelings of sadness or guilt may have a negative impact on your feelings for your partner or your sexual well-being. If you feel the need to receive counselling, talk to your GP who can provide you with a list of recognised counsellors in your area, or contact Relate.*

Fertility

A relatively high proportion of couples have difficulty conceiving a baby, and it can be a very upsetting experience. There are, however, a number of ways you can improve your chances of getting pregnant.

For example, make love at least every other day, especially in the three days either side of ovulation, which is your most fertile time. You can use ovulation prediction kits or tests to check whether you have ovulated. Stopping smoking or reducing your alcohol intake (for both you and your partner) may make a difference. However, there is no truth in the myth that making love in any particular position can enhance your chances of getting pregnant.

There is also much that can be done medically to assist couples in conceiving. These methods are covered below.

Fertility worries

Q *My partner wants us to try for a baby now, although I would rather wait a few years as I am only 21. He is 25 and reckons that we shouldn't wait too long because sperm counts are falling all the time due to environmental poisoning. Is this true? Will four or five more years make any difference?*

A There is a great deal of debate about whether male fertility is declining as a result of modern environmental hazards. There have been various studies, but their results conflict. According to semen samples collected from 1,385 Los Angeles men between 1994 and 1997 and compared with samples in a 1951 study, men today produce just as many sperm as their grandfathers did. However, other evidence suggests that sperm counts are falling, and the role that drugs, smoking, infections and stress play in fertility, both male and female, is still unclear.

However, the majority of men are still producing sperm in sufficient numbers and of good enough quality to have no problem with fertility. Treatments such as chemotherapy can affect fertility (see Chapter 4), but if your partner is only 25, has not had chemotherapy or serious illness, or surgery that may affect his fertility, he should not worry unduly. Any fears about his sperm count are probably unfounded and are not a good reason to rush into pregnancy too soon. If he is worried about his own sperm count, he can arrange through his GP to get a semen sample analysed at the local hospital lab.

Difficulty conceiving

Q *I have been trying to get pregnant for nearly a year now, with no success. Could I have a hormone imbalance? I have read somewhere that this can be a cause of problems with conceiving.*

A If your periods are regular, then any hormonal imbalance you may have is highly unlikely to be affecting your fertility.

You can find out whether you ovulate by buying a special fertility thermometer (available from the chemist) and taking your temperature every morning to detect the change in average temperature that occurs around the time of ovulation. However, this method is now being superseded by ovulation prediction kits, also available from pharmacists: they are more expensive but are very accurate at showing whether and when you have ovulated. Equally effective is a blood test, which your GP can do for you on day 21 of your cycle (i.e. 21 days after the first day of your last period) to see whether your hormone levels suggest you have ovulated that month.

Remember that it takes, on average, one year for a normal couple to conceive a baby. However, if you have been trying for longer than a year, or if you are over 35, have never been pregnant or have some other reason to worry about your or your partner's fertility, then go to your GP and ask for further advice.

Q *My wife and I have been trying for a baby for nearly a year now. We are both in our mid-thirties and are both healthy with no particular medical problems. We desperately want to have children but are rather reluctant to get involved with doctors and lots of tests and treatments. Do you think we should?*

A Your reluctance is quite understandable. After all, making love and making a baby is a very private thing that you share with your wife, and the idea of having to discuss it with a doctor is rather daunting. You will almost certainly be asked to produce a sperm sample, and this thought alone puts many men off seeking help. However, it would make sense for you and your wife to bite the bullet and make an appointment to see your GP together. Your wife will have blood tests and will be asked about her periods and any previous pregnancies, and you will both be asked about operations, illnesses, medication and whether you are managing to make love in the fertile period – which lasts for five days or so, starting around ten days after your wife's period starts. Further tests can be organised by a fertility specialist, often a gynaecologist.

Q *What causes infertility? We have been trying for a baby for six months, to no avail, and are beginning to get worried.*

A It takes the average couple a year to conceive. Of those who have difficulty in conceiving:

- in about four out of ten couples, the woman has a specific problem
- in another four out of ten couples, the man has a specific problem
- in the remaining two out of ten couples, there are problems with both the man and woman, or no cause can be found.

The most common reasons for fertility problems are as follows.

- The woman does not produce an egg (ovulate) regularly or at all. Many women find that their periods stop for a while if they lose or gain a lot of weight suddenly, or if they travel, change job or are otherwise stressed. Periods normally restart on their own once normal weight is regained or the stress subsides. (Although ovulation is not necessarily synchronised with periods, in practice the latter is a good indication of the former.) Stopping the contraceptive pill is said not to interfere with fertility, but some women find that their cycles take a while to get back to their normal pattern. The drug clomiphene (Clomid) is sometimes prescribed to stimulate ovulation.
- Blockage of the Fallopian tubes, which lead from the ovaries to the womb. These tubes need to be entirely unconstricted to allow free passage of the egg, but blockages can occur because of previous infections or operations. An ectopic pregnancy, appendicitis, infections which have spread up from the vagina and womb (pelvic inflammatory disease) or inflammation from endometriosis (see Chapter 5 for more about these), can all make the tubes stick together or be plastered down by 'adhesions' – bands of tissue that form when there is inflammation or infection. An operation to unblock the tubes may be attempted, but IVF (see below) can often offer more hope.
- A condition called polycystic ovary syndrome (PCOS – see Chapter 5). PCOS does not necessarily cause problems, but it can cause a hormone imbalance with excess male hormones (androgens), resulting in acne, infertility and facial hair. The condition is more common in overweight women. Losing excess

weight, treatment with drugs that stimulate ovulation, e.g. clomiphene (Clomid), or an operation to disrupt the ovaries in order to stimulate them to work, can all be successful.

- An obstruction in the womb. This is a rare cause of infertility. As part of the normal investigation for infertility a gynaecologist will look into the womb with a hysteroscope (telescope) to ensure there is no problem.
- Early menopause. Some women go into the menopause before the age of 40, and this means that their ovaries will stop working and will not produce eggs. The only hope for pregnancy in these cases is by using donor eggs (see below).
- Various hormone disorders (in both men and women), which can prevent ovulation and conception. A GP or gynaecologist can take a blood sample to test for various hormone levels, and treatment depends on finding a specific cause.
- The man's sperm may not be healthy enough to fertilise the egg. As part of the investigations for infertility, he will be asked to produce a semen sample, by masturbating, which will be analysed in the laboratory. In the past, men with low sperm counts would be told there was nothing that could be done. Treatment still presents a great challenge, but semen can now be treated in the laboratory to improve the chances of pregnancy. Techniques like ICSI (see below) offer hope. Occasionally there may be a blockage in the tube that carries sperm from the testicle, and an operation to retrieve sperm from the exit to the testicle can now be done without a general anaesthetic.

Assisted conception

Q *We have had all the tests for infertility and no cause has been found. I am now 38 and the gynaecologist has advised IVF. I am trying to find out more about this and other techniques. Can you help?*

A **In-vitro fertilisation (IVF)** is when the eggs are fertilised by sperm outside the body (in a test tube) and then placed in the womb. Drugs are first given to the woman to stimulate the ovaries to produce several eggs instead of the usual one. The eggs are taken from the ovaries using a vaginal scanner, which is passed up the vagina and has a fine needle attached to retrieve the eggs. A sedative

179

and painkiller are used, but a general anaesthetic is not necessary. A sperm sample is supplied by the man, and is mixed with the eggs. If the sperm fertilise the eggs, the fertilised eggs (embryos) are put in the woman's womb a couple of days later, in a procedure similar to having a smear test. A maximum of three embryos are usually replaced. Hormone pessaries (which are put in the vagina) or injections keep the lining of the womb primed to accept the embryo.

Possible problems with IVF include a one-in-four chance of having twins and a one-in-20 chance of triplets, if pregnancy occurs. Minor problems, such as sickness, headaches and feeling irritable, may be due to the drugs used to stimulate the ovaries. They may sometimes be too sensitive to the hormones and produce numerous eggs. This can cause vomiting, lower abdominal pain and bloating, and occasionally leads to hospital admission. There is also an increased chance of an ectopic pregnancy, but the ultrasound scan, which is done if a pregnancy test is positive, should pick this up at an early stage.

Gamete intrafallopian transfer (GIFT) is an alternative technique, though used less often nowadays. Drugs to stimulate the ovaries are given, as for IVF. The difference is that the woman has a general anaesthetic and, using a laparoscope (telescope) inserted into the abdomen, the eggs are collected and eggs and sperm are put into the Fallopian tube, where they are left to fertilise. Obviously, only women with normal, unblocked tubes can have this done.

Pronuclear stage embryo transfer (PROST) is similar to IVF. The fertilised eggs are put into the Fallopian tubes using a laparoscope, rather than into the womb through the vagina.

Intracytoplasmic sperm injection (ICSI) offers hope for men with very few active sperm who cannot fertilise eggs with IVF. A single sperm is injected directly into an egg which has been retrieved from the woman, as with IVF.

Artificial insemination by husband (AIH) uses a syringe to introduce the sperm into the woman's cervix at the time in the month when she is ovulating (this is usually exactly 14 days before the next period is due). If the sperm are few, slow-moving or have many abnormalities, the semen can first be processed to select the most active sperm.

Donor insemination (DI) uses sperm from donors, usually from students, which has been screened for sexually transmitted diseases, including HIV, and genetically inherited diseases. The sperm donor has no legal rights or obligations. As with AIH, the sperm are introduced into the cervix at the time of month when the woman is ovulating.

Intrauterine/insemination (IUI) introduces the sperm straight into the womb, through the vagina and cervix. The sperm are specially treated and the woman may be given drugs to help her to produce more than one egg in order to increase the chances of pregnancy.

Egg donation is the only option for women who are not producing eggs. The eggs can be fertilised by the woman's partner's sperm, and the embryo can be placed in the womb while hormones are used to keep the pregnancy going.

Which technique for which problem?

Problem	Techniques that may be suitable
Sperm too few or too slow	ICSI, DI or IVF
Woman's body 'hostile' to sperm, e.g. makes antibodies against sperm or cervix produces barrier to sperm	IUI or IVF
Problems with intercourse, e.g. spasm in vagina (vaginismus) or male impotence	AIH, IUI, DI or IVF
Unexplained infertility	AIH, IUI or IVF
Poor-quality eggs and lack of response to IVF	ICSI
Sperm cannot get to egg, e.g. blocked Fallopian tubes due to previous sterilisation of woman, endometriosis or previous ectopic pregnancies	IVF
Irregular ovulation	IVF
Woman wants to conceive without intercourse with a man, e.g. in a lesbian couple	DI

GIFT or PROST techniques may be offered in place of IVF, so long as the Fallopian tubes are normal.

Dealing with childlessness

Q *My husband and I have been through the infertility mill. We have had two attempts at IVF and we don't think we can stand the emotional or financial strain of going through it again. Although the experts can find no particular underlying cause, we are becoming resigned to the fact that we will probably never have children. I feel so terribly sad about this and I really don't know how I will cope. Can you offer any advice?*

A It can be extremely hard to come to terms with childlessness. The yearning for children is a very strong and fundamental one, but, as you have discovered, fertility treatments are not always successful.

If you decide to give IVF another go, look at the information from the Human Fertilisation and Embryology Authority (HFEA),★ which assesses the different centres. It ensures that all UK treatment clinics that offer in-vitro fertilisation (IVF), donor insemination (DI), or store eggs, sperm or embryos, conform to high medical and professional standards. It collects data about the treatments and provides detailed advice and information to the public.

Once you decide to stop all fertility treatments, you will almost certainly consider adopting or fostering a child. The Adoption Information Line★ is an invaluable resource: it provides details of regional services and adoption agencies as well as information about fostering.

Of course, these options may not work out for you, and you may have to resign yourselves to life as a couple without children. In that case you can expect to go through a painful process which is very similar to bereavement after a death. After a feeling of numbness, you will probably experience anger – which may be directed against each other, health professionals, or close friends and family. This is often followed by intense sadness and mourning for your lost opportunities. After time, however, resolution and acceptance usually prevail. There may be poignant moments which will be particularly hard to bear, but most childless couples do come to accept their situation and feel that they can go on to live happy and fulfilled lives.

There is good ongoing support from an organisation called CHILD (National Infertility Support Network).★ Another excellent organisation is MoreToLife,★ which is dedicated to providing support to those involuntarily childless for whom fertility treatment is no longer a consideration. It offers help in exploring all that a life without children has to offer, while accepting people's need to grieve and to have support in adjusting to a different kind of future.

The menopause

'Menopause' simply means the end of the menses, or periods. The underlying reason for this is that the ovaries stop functioning. This means they stop producing eggs, but also that the levels of oestrogen and progesterone fall. It is the fall in oestrogen that causes some of the problems that women experience after the menopause, such as hot flushes and a dry vagina. The loss of oestrogen also means the loss of its protection against, for example, the onset of osteoporosis and heart disease.

The menopause need not be a big deal, but many find it very troubling. Most choose to take no special medication or precautions to alleviate its effects, some take nutritional supplements, and some opt for hormone replacement therapy (HRT). Each woman going through the menopause will need to weigh up the pros and cons of these options to make her own decision.

Early menopause

Q *I am in my mid-thirties and seem to be experiencing a complete change in menstruation. I used to have very heavy periods, but now I get just one full day of extremely light bleeding every month, followed by a little spotting for two or three days. In addition to this my emotions are all over the place: there are moments, leading up to a period, when I feel incredibly weepy, which is not at all like me. I have also been having night sweats. Surely this is not the start of the menopause? What do you think?*

A It certainly is possible to go into the menopause younger than the average age of 50. Interestingly, if you smoke, you may get the menopause two years earlier than average, though this would not account for your periods becoming scanty in your thirties. The first signs of impending menopause are often:

- hot flushes
- night sweats

- dry vagina, which makes you prone to urine infections and may make sex painful
- changes to your normal periods – lighter or heavier; more or less frequent
- mood changes, especially just before or during a period.

However, it is important to be aware that you cannot attribute everything that happens to you between now and the age of 60 to the menopause. So if you are getting very tense and irritable, especially around period times, perhaps you need some specific stress-managing techniques – a yoga class once a week or some reorganisation at home to take some of the strain off you.

Your GP can do a blood test (FSH) which measures the level of hormone that controls the ovaries. When the menopause occurs, the ovaries stop working and the FSH levels go up. If your FSH is, say, 20 now and goes up to 35 in six months' time, it suggests that you are indeed building up to the menopause. As part of the same blood test, your thyroid hormone can be measured, since an overactive thyroid (see Chapter 1) makes periods scanty. You can also be checked for anaemia, which might be making you feel excessively tired.

If blood tests and the pattern of your periods suggest that you are approaching the menopause, you will want to think carefully about hormone replacement therapy (HRT – see below), which may well have many advantages for you.

Do not forget that you cannot assume you are no longer fertile until you have not had a period for over a year and tests suggest that this is due to the menopause. If in doubt, and if you do not want to get pregnant, err on the side of caution and use contraception!

Post-menopausal bleeding

Q *I have been going through the menopause for the past year, and thought that my periods had finally stopped. However, I have recently experienced some more bleeding, and wonder if this is anything to worry about?*

A If you have any vaginal bleeding after the menopause, you need to get it checked out. This means any vaginal bleeding that occurs more than six months after your last period. (Although the menopause occurs when you have your last menstrual period (LMP), you cannot know for sure that it is your last until a full year has elapsed.) Women often tend to dismiss the bleeding, thinking it is just another, rather late period – and indeed it sometimes is. It is also very commonly due to breakthrough bleeding, if you are on HRT.

However, in 10–20 per cent of cases, vaginal bleeding after the menopause is due to an underlying cancer, usually of the lining of the womb (endometrial cancer) and so should never be ignored. Other causes of the bleeding can be sore, dry cracks in the vagina, which develop after the menopause because of the lack of oestrogen; non-cancerous growths in the cervix or womb (e.g. fibroids or polyps); or injury (e.g. from over-enthusiastic sex). Occasionally, the blood is not coming from the vagina at all but from piles in your back passage or is due to a urine infection.

Your GP will want to do a vaginal examination, blood tests for anaemia, smear test and urine test, and to arrange an ultrasound scan. Referral to a gynaecologist to look into your womb and take a small sample from its lining will be arranged unless it is certain that there is a harmless explanation for the bleeding. In most cases the cause is harmless, but it is always worth taking seriously and getting checked.

Hormone replacement therapy (HRT)

Pros and cons of HRT

Q *I am 49 and my doctor tells me I am entering the menopause. She has provided me with lots of information about HRT, which seems to be something of a mixed blessing. What do you think – is it advisable to take it?*

A The menopause means that your ovaries no longer produce oestrogen, so levels of the hormone fall and this leads to a range of potential problems. HRT replaces the oestrogen. Whether or not you want to keep your oestrogen levels up or let nature take its course is entirely up to you: there is no right or wrong answer, but it may help to summarise the pros and cons of HRT for you.

On the positive side:

- it is great for hot flushes, sweats, and vaginal dryness
- it is the best way of preventing osteoporosis (bone thinning). The longer you take HRT for, the more years of protection you 'buy' your bones
- there is some evidence to suggest that it protects against heart disease and Alzheimer's dementia

- some women say it helps mood disturbances and lack of concentration. However, obviously it is not a panacea and it does not guarantee eternal youth.

On the negative side:

- it slightly increases your risk of getting a thrombosis. You cannot take HRT if you have had a thrombosis, and the incidence of thrombosis among women using HRT is 3 in 10,000 per year, compared to 1 in 10,000 per year among those not using it
- there is a possible increase in the risk of breast cancer after five to ten years of use (see below). There is no evidence that using HRT for less than five years significantly increases your risk of breast cancer – but it is a worry that puts a lot of women off HRT

Is HRT for you?

Ask yourself the following questions to see whether you would benefit from HRT.

- Am I suffering from the menopause? (Hot flushes, night sweats, breast tenderness?)
- Am I at risk of osteoporosis? (The following are risk factors for osteoporosis: menopause before the age of 45, a first-degree female relative with osteoporosis, smoking, having a high alcohol or caffeine intake, having had prolonged anorexia, using steroids or thyroids long-term, being of small build, being of Asian or Caucasian origin.)
- Am I at risk of heart disease? (The following are risk factors for heart disease: menopause before the age of 45, a first-degree relative with heart disease, smoking, inherited high levels of cholesterol, high blood pressure, diabetes, obesity causing diabetes or an increase in high blood pressure. See Chapter 1.)
- Am I at low risk for breast cancer? (i.e. No previous benign lumps whose cells showed a pre-cancerous abnormality, no first-degree female relative with breast cancer. See Chapter 5.)
- Am I at low risk for thrombosis? (i.e. No previous thrombosis, no strong family history of thrombosis, not obese, immobile, or a smoker.)

- there are 'minor' side-effects in around 15 per cent of users. These include breast tenderness, weight gain, nausea, headaches, itchy skin, rashes, mood swings and fluid retention
- with most preparations you will get a monthly bleed. A three-monthly bleed or no bleed at all is possible with some preparations
- abnormal vaginal bleeding, usually spotting throughout the cycle, can be a problem and needs to be investigated if it persists.

Which type of HRT?

Q *I would like to take HRT but was rather bemused when my GP asked me whether I'd rather try a patch, tablet, implant or vaginal cream. What is the difference, and which type is best?*

A It depends on your needs and your own menopausal symptoms. For example, if you have a problem with vaginal dryness, you could use a vaginal cream. If you have had a hysterectomy, you will be able to take oestrogen on its own, whether as a tablet, patch, vaginal cream or pessary, or as an implant under the skin. But if you still have a womb, oestrogen on its own can lead to endometrial cancer (cancer of the lining of the womb) so in order to protect it you need to take progestogens (the generic name for progesterone-like hormones) for at least ten days a month in addition to the oestrogen. These are known as combined preparations.

If you have had a period in the last 12 months or are younger than 54, you will be prescribed a preparation that gives you monthly 'periods'. But if you are well into the menopause – i.e. you have not had a period for over a year or are older than 54, you can use a preparation that does not give you 'periods'.

Patches allow the hormones to go straight into your bloodstream, bypassing your stomach. But some women find that they irritate the skin and some say they find wearing a patch rather embarrassing. Taking a daily tablet, or two tablets in some preparations, is convenient for some women but does not suit everyone.

Having an implant under the skin requires a visit to a clinic or doctor's surgery and can sometimes cause pain, bleeding and infection. However, once it is in it lasts for up to six months, so some women consider it to be worth the discomfort or inconvenience.

Long-term HRT

Q *I am very happy to be on HRT – it suits me and I am reluctant to stop it. But my GP has said that since I have been on it for ten years now, I should come off it. Do I have to?*

A Taking HRT is a question of balancing the pros and cons of it for you as an individual (see above). The concern about long-term use arises from the current evidence that suggests that after five years of continuous use of HRT, there is a small increase in the risk of breast cancer. This is more marked after ten years of use. As ongoing studies report their findings, this information may change.

You have a 1-in-22 chance of developing breast cancer between the ages of 50 and 70 if you have never taken HRT, a 1-in-19 chance after 10 years of use and a 1-in-17 chance after 15 years of HRT. Whether you continue taking HRT or not, you would be well advised to attend for three-yearly mammograms from the age of 50 and to be aware of your breasts and report any lumps or changes that you find.

You are considered to be at relatively low risk of breast cancer if neither you nor members of your family have had it. You may have a strong reason for wanting to take HRT – such as horrible hot flushes, a dry vagina, or a high risk of osteoporosis, heart disease or dementia – and for these reasons you may be prepared to put up with a slight increase in the risk of breast cancer.

(See Chapter 5 for more about breast cancer.)

Natural alternatives to HRT

Q *I am entering the menopause and suffering from night sweats and hot flushes. However, I am very reluctant to take HRT as I don't want to be putting artificial hormones into my body on a regular basis. Are there any natural alternatives?*

A Yes, there are lots of options, although you may find it comforting to know, with regard to your hot flushes and night sweats, that the average duration of these unpleasant symptoms is 18 months – so they certainly will not go on for ever. In the meantime it makes sense to avoid situations which make you flushed naturally, such as overheated rooms, being too warmly dressed, drinking alcohol and eating spicy foods. There are also natural methods that you can try to combat your menopausal symptoms:

- you can boost your oestrogen levels by eating natural oestrogens – phytoestrogens, found in soy and linseed – or trying a supplement, available from health food shops. These may be very beneficial in combating the adverse effects of the menopause
- vitamin B6 and evening primrose oil may help mood swings
- the non-hormonal drug clonidine, which is available on prescription, can prevent hot flushes, although it is not always effective
- the value of natural progesterone skin cream remains unproven, but some women swear by it.

You can also use natural methods to protect against the other long-term risks that increase with the menopause. These are as follows.

- To prevent osteoporosis – a high-calcium diet (e.g. 1,000mg/day of calcium), regular exercise, and not smoking helps to keep bones strong. You can also have a bone-density scan every year to check for osteoporosis. Non-hormonal medication is available to treat the condition, including calcium, calcitonin or bisphosphonates.
- To prevent heart disease – a low-fat diet including oily fish, regular exercise and no smoking. Vitamins C, E and beta-carotene, found in the diet and also available as supplements, may also offer protection against heart disease and breast cancer.

Chapter 7

Digestion and bottoms

Most of us cringe at the thought of having to discuss bottom- or gut-related concerns with a doctor. But an itchy anus, excess wind, abdominal bloating or blood on the toilet paper when we wipe ourselves are extremely common problems. Most of these symptoms are caused by harmless conditions rather than any serious underlying disease. They can all be helped, and it is a shame to suffer and fret unnecessarily.

In addition to these worries, this chapter looks at widespread complaints such as heartburn and irritable bowel syndrome, as well as more unusual ones such as difficulty in swallowing. It identifies common causes of troubling symptoms and discusses the possibility of serious conditions, including bowel cancer. This will help you to determine when you should see a doctor, and when you will be able to treat yourself.

The glossary of medical terms will demystify what your doctor might say, and help you to overcome your embarrassment if you feel more comfortable using medical language.

Difficulty swallowing

Q *What is 'globus'? My doctor says my girlfriend may have it. We know very little about it other than that it is a condition of the throat, and we are quite worried. Can you tell us any more?*

A A 'globus' implies that your girlfriend has difficulty swallowing but that no physical cause can be found to account for it. It suggests that the cause is largely a psychological problem. However, that does not mean that the problem is not real. In many people difficulty swallowing properly is initially caused by a physical condition. They may have, say, acid reflux from the stomach (see page 194) or a bad dose of tonsillitis. That problem usually passes on its own and without any particular treatment, but it may leave behind a persistent fear of swallowing.

If the doctor has ruled out physical causes of painful swallowing such as narrowing of the oesophagus owing to acid reflux or even cancer, you have to find out what the reason for the globus is. You may find it hard to get practical help for your girlfriend. It might be useful for you and her to book a double appointment with your GP and forewarn him or her that you would like to discuss the whole problem. He or she can look through your girlfriend's notes and perhaps speak to any specialists she may have seen at a hospital.

Glossary

Abdomen   Stomach/belly

Anus   Back passage

Barium enema   A chemical inserted into your anus which shows up on an X-ray

Colon   The large bowel

Colonoscopy   An examination by a camera of the entire colon via an instrument inserted into your back passage

Colostomy   Surgical procedure to open a section of bowel on to the surface of the skin. The bowel contents can then be collected into a bag attached around the opening

Digital rectal examination   An examination of your anus using a gloved finger

Endoscopy   Examination of oesophagus, stomach and first part of small intestine, using a tube pushed down into your stomach

Faeces   Bowel movement (stool or 'poo')

Flatus   Farts

Gastro-enterologist   Specialist in digestive problems, but not a surgeon

Haemorrhoids   Piles

Mucus   Slime

Oesophagus   Food pipe/gullet. The tube between mouth and stomach

Sigmoidoscopy   An examination of your lower bowel using a telescope inserted through the anus

Suppository   Medication which is inserted into your back passage

A full and frank explanation of the tests and the results may help to alleviate any residual fears she has. Then she can slowly try to regain confidence in swallowing normally. Some specific counselling may be needed.

Q *I have great difficulty with pills and tablets. I have tried swallowing them with and without water, but they just get stuck in my throat, and I often end up choking. Consequently I avoid taking tablets if I can help it, and I now have a mental block about them – they just fill me with horror. I am embarrassed to mention it to my doctor. Can you suggest why I should have this problem and what I could do to solve it?*

A Being unable to swallow tablets is quite a common problem. Clearly, if you have difficulty swallowing food or drink, you may have an underlying condition that needs urgent investigation. But if the situation is confined to tablets and everything else slips down your throat smoothly, you really do not need to worry. It is possible that your fear of swallowing tablets arises from previous unpleasant experiences with them – being forced to swallow huge tablets, say, or having a bitter-tasting pill starting to dissolve in your mouth before you can swallow it whole. If you want to overcome your antipathy to tablets and pills, try a tiny, coated pill such as a multivitamin pill made for children, to show yourself that you can do it if you really try. If you are ever prescribed vital medication by a doctor you can either ask for a syrup or soluble tablet if they are available, or speak to the pharmacist about finding a formulation that suits you, as the size of tablets varies with brand and dose.

Q *I have had difficulty with eating and swallowing for two years now. At first doctors prescribed antibiotics for stomach upsets, then they said they believed the symptoms were psychological and gave me antidepressants. Now I have been told that my oesophagus is closed over and that I have achalasia, often preventing food and liquids from entering my stomach for many hours. Can you tell me more about it?*

A Achalasia is a fairly rare condition but it is eminently treatable. No one really understands why it happens, but in some people the waves of muscular contraction (peristalsis) that normally propel food down the oesophagus do not work, and the opening from the oesophagus into the stomach does not open to let food in. This leads to difficulty in swallowing fluids and solids, regurgitation of undigested food shortly after a meal, heartburn after eating and weight loss in more severe cases. Because the condition is caused by a mechanical problem, it does not get better on its own and may get worse. Surgery is often the only long-term option.

You could be offered one of three procedures to treat the achalasia. Injections of botulinum toxin (a drug that weakens the strong muscle contractions) into the muscle at the opening of the stomach, via a tube inserted through the mouth (endoscopy), works well but the effects do not last long and it is usually offered only to elderly or frail people. Cutting the muscle at the opening of the stomach (myomectomy) is successful in 80 to 90 per cent of cases and is safe, but it may cause discomfort and is a fairly major operation. The third option, inserting a deflated balloon down the oesophagus via an endoscope, then inflating it to stretch the opening into the stomach, is slightly less likely to succeed (it has a success rate of about 60 per cent) but it causes less discomfort and patients recover more quickly. You should discuss the pros and cons of these different procedures with your surgeon before making your decision.

Mucus in the throat

Q *I have a throat problem that just will not go away. It feels like I have a lot of mucus that I can't get rid of, no matter what I try. I am constantly swallowing and it is making me feel very sick. It is particularly bad when I try to get to sleep. My life is very stressful at the moment – I have a child who is ill – and I am worried about myself. Is there anything you could suggest to help me?*

A The discomfort in your throat and nausea when you try to sleep suggest that you might be suffering from acid reflux (see below). With all the worries you must have about your child, it would not be surprising if your stomach were producing excess acid. If an antacid such as sodium alginate (Gaviscon) gets rid of the unpleasant sensation, you have your answer. To prevent a recurrence of the reflux, cut out spicy foods and alcohol, eat small, frequent meals, lose excess weight and sleep with an extra pillow. Managing your stress levels must be a real challenge: try to put some time aside for yourself to help you cope, whether that means going to a yoga class, having a night out with friends or speaking to a trained third party. (See Chapter 2 for more about anxiety and stress.)

If the Gaviscon does not help at all, you may want to ask your GP to refer you to a gastro-enterologist for further tests to rule out less likely but potentially more dangerous causes of your problems, such as a stomach ulcer or cancer of the stomach or oesophagus.

Acid reflux

Q *I have started getting the most awful heartburn, often in the middle of the night. During the day I burp frequently, sometimes without warning. The other day I let out a huge burp in a crowded lift at work, and wanted to die of embarrassment. I feel terribly bloated and cannot do up any of my trousers or skirts. I have tried drinking a glass of milk at night, and hot water after my meals, but these measures have not helped at all. Can you offer any advice?*

A You may find it comforting to know that 40 per cent of the British population get heartburn, also known as acid regurgitation or reflux (or in medi-speak as gastro-oesophageal reflux disease or GORD). The problem occurs because the sphincter that lies at the bottom of the oesophagus relaxes temporarily and lets acid from the stomach flow back up the food pipe. The acid causes burning behind the breastbone as it washes up the oesophagus, an acid taste in the mouth and excess gas, which accounts for the burping and bloating. Only a third of people with reflux ever see a doctor about it, which is a shame because effective treatments do exist.

The first step is to cut down on excessive alcohol, fatty foods and smoking, all of which can exacerbate the reflux. A lot of people find out the hard way which foods to avoid: tomatoes, citrus fruits, pickles and hot curries are common culprits. Stress triggers heartburn in some people, so stress-management techniques such as yoga may be very effective. Drugs that neutralise acid, such as sodium alginate (Gaviscon), and others that block acid, such as cimetidine (Tagamet) or ranitidine (Zantac), can be bought over the counter. But the drugs that switch off acid production in the stomach, such as omeprazole (Losec), are available only on prescription, so a visit to the GP may be helpful. If you do not get better with treatment, or have additional symptoms such as unexplained weight loss, difficulty swallowing or passing blood in your stool, you will be referred for an endoscopy – an examination of the inside of your oesophagus and stomach.

Persistent sickness

Q *I have had a repeated sickness bug over the last year – every three months or so I get 24 hours of vomiting and nausea followed by 'flu-like symptoms. Could each bout be linked with the same dormant bug? Is there anything I can do to prevent this from happening again?*

A Bugs do not usually lie dormant in our bodies. Our immune systems are designed to fight each bug as it invades our body, so each time we are exposed to a new bug we may get ill again. Exposure to some bugs, e.g. the chickenpox virus, confers lifelong immunity so once you have had the illness, you should not catch it again.

Experiencing 24 hours of nausea, vomiting and feeling unwell could have a number of causes. If you get a headache with it, perhaps it is a migraine (see Chapter 10). If you are dizzy and have hearing loss, you may have Menière's disease, which affects the inner ear. If you are being exposed to bugs that cause stomach upsets (e.g. a bug called cryptosporidium in the water supply), it seems odd that it happens only every few months and you are well in between.

Some women have similar symptoms just before a period. Keeping a detailed record of when the symptoms occur and what you had eaten in the 24 hours preceding the attack may help to shed light on the cause.

If you are not losing weight, feel well between bouts and have no blood loss in the stool or other worrying features, your symptoms are unlikely to be caused by any dangerous condition, but you should certainly seek medical advice.

Abdominal pain

Q *I have a sharp pain that appears and disappears in the lower right-hand side of my abdomen. It has been sore to touch on occasions. Is this a sign of appendicitis? Could I have a grumbling appendix? Every time I go to the doctor, the pain disappears and I am too embarrassed to go again. Should I pursue the subject with my doctor?*

A You are quite right that the lower right-hand side of your abdomen is where your appendix is. The appendix comes off the last bit of the small intestine, where it joins the large intestine. The small and large intestines are connected via a balloon-like bit of bowel called the caecum which has very stretchy walls and where gas often collects. People who get a lot of bloating and wind often experience a sharp pain in this lower right-hand corner of the abdomen as the caecum gets distended with gas. Appendicitis can cause the same kind of pain, but it tends to be accompanied by constipation and a slight fever. Moreover, the pain gets increasingly severe until you really cannot put up with it. Appendicitis does occur in adult life but is relatively uncommon compared with the problem of excess wind, which may be part of irritable bowel syndrome (see below). A 'grumbling appendix', on the other hand, is something that surgeons do not really believe exists.

If bloating and gas are the problem, try:

- eating a medium-fibre (not high-fibre) diet
- drinking lots of fluids
- avoiding gas-forming foods, such as baked beans
- doing aerobic exercise every day to get bowels moving
- having mebeverine (Colofac) or hyoscine (Buscopan) or charcoal preparations.

Hernia

Q *I think I may be suffering from some kind of looseness of the stomach wall. My abdomen sticks out above my belly button, which is causing me a great deal of distress as it is very noticeable under clothes. Is surgery the only option – as I have been told by my GP – or are there other ways of dealing with the problem, such as exercising or dieting?*

A It sounds as though you may have a hernia – a protrusion of the abdominal contents through a weakness in the abdominal wall. These weaknesses can occur in different parts of the abdominal wall. Swellings in the groin are inguinal or femoral hernias, protruding belly buttons (usually seen in young babies) are umbilical hernias, and bulges above the belly button are para-umbilical or epigastric hernias. The abdominal wall weakness may be an inherited condition, or it could have been caused by an operation or injury. Often the weakness has no obvious cause. Hernias rarely disappear on their own and tend to get bigger rather than smaller over several years. An operation involving darning the abdominal wall or sewing a patch over the weakened area is often advised, as there is a risk of loops of bowel getting trapped in the hernia, which can be disastrous. Some hernias are more dangerous than others but your GP will certainly want to refer you to a surgeon for a specialist opinion.

Excess wind and bloating

> **Possible causes of wind**
>
> **Gas-forming foods** (e.g. cabbage, beans)
>
> **Irritable bowel syndrome (IBS)**
>
> An underlying gut disease, such as **Crohn's disease** or **ulcerative colitis** (see below) – however, these also have additional symptoms such as weight loss, fever and blood in the stool

Irritable bowel syndrome

Q *I have terrible wind, which makes me feel bloated and generates smelly farts that I cannot control. I have been told that I have irritable bowel syndrome. I am not sure what this means – could you please enlighten me?*

A Although irritable bowel syndrome (IBS) is very common indeed, its causes are not known. The treatment for it therefore involves alleviating the symptoms.

The symptoms of IBS, which can come and go, include:

* abdominal pain
* bloated abdomen
* diarrhoea and/or constipation
* passing clear 'slime' from the back passage
* feeling the needing to pass a motion, even when there is none to pass
* lethargy, backache, or pain on passing urine.

In some people the symptoms are aggravated by stress, stomach upsets and specific foods.

It seems that the whole of the gut is affected in IBS – for some unknown reason, the gut muscle goes into spasm. In the upper part, this causes indigestion, burping and discomfort. In the lower part, IBS can cause lower abdominal pain, diarrhoea or constipation.

Q *I know I have IBS but am not sure how to help myself. Do you have any suggestions?*

A You need to recognise that IBS is a specific condition that will tend to come and go. It is reassuring to know that however bad the symptoms are, they are not dangerous.

For constipation try eating a varied, fibre-rich diet and drinking plenty of fluids. However, some people's IBS is made worse by eating more fibre, especially wheat bran. Laxative preparations may also help but can worsen bloating. Exercise can help to relieve constipation.

Crohn's disease

Crohn's disease is a chronic (long-term) disease, which causes inflammation of parts of the digestive tract. Any part, from the mouth to the anus and along the length of the bowel can be affected, and if the bowel wall is affected it becomes red, swollen and ulcerated. The cause of Crohn's disease is unknown. There can be an inherited tendency, smoking increases the risk, and there may be dietary or viral causes, but the full picture is still not understood.

Crohn's can result in bouts of diarrhoea, failure to absorb foods, abdominal pains, fever, weight loss, bleeding from the back passage and ill health. More rarely, severe complications such as obstruction of the bowels can arise. An elemental diet, in which all but a few simple foods are banned, can help when there is a flare-up. Fish oils may help prevent recurrences, steroids (both orally and rectally) can help symptoms, and antibiotics may be useful to heal the fissures (painful cracks around the back passage) if they are infected. In bad flare-ups, resting the gut and giving all fluids and nutrients intravenously may be necessary. Surgery is sometimes needed for complications such as abscesses and obstruction.

Treat pain with an anti-spasmodic drug, most of which are available over the counter, such as peppermint-oil capsules (Colpermin), mebeverine (Colofac) and alverine (Spasmonal). If one does not work, try another.

For severe diarrhoea try loperamide (Imodium, Arret, Diocalm Ultra), available over the counter, or co-phenotrope (Lomotil), available on prescription.

Try to maintain a positive approach, managing symptoms as and when they occur.

You could try an exclusion diet – a specially tailored diet which excludes many foods and introduces them back one by one, and which may help diarrhoea. However, such a diet is best supervised by a dietician. Some GP surgeries have a dietician on site.

Gut-directed hypnotherapy, which allows the IBS sufferer to focus on the gut and learn to control symptoms, can be very valuable. It is not widely available, but it is worth asking a GP if the local

---

Ulcerative colitis

Ulcerative colitis (UC) is similar to Crohn's disease. However, it is more common and is usually (though not always) milder than Crohn's, and tends to affect a continuous section of the large bowel rather than causing the intermittent patches of disease that occur throughout the gut in Crohn's. Outside the tropics, UC is the most common cause of prolonged bloody diarrhoea (i.e. lasting more than seven days). The cause of the disease is unknown, although there may be an inherited tendency in some cases. The symptoms include diarrhoea, abdominal pain and rectal bleeding.

Weight loss, fever and ill health can also be problems in more severe cases. Flare-ups are treated with drugs, usually oral and rectal steroids, and long-term treatment with drugs such as sulfasalazine (Salazopyrin) are advised to try to prevent recurrences. Complications in severe cases can include dehydration, internal bleeding, bowel perforation and an increased risk of bowel cancer (10 per cent of those with UC for over 25 years may develop bowel cancer). Surgery may be required for complications.

Most people with UC are not incapacitated by it and many have long periods of time with no problems at all.

specialists (gastro-enterologists) offer it. General hypnotherapy is not as effective usually.

Psychotherapy can also be helpful. Again, availability on the NHS is extremely limited.

Q *I have been told I have IBS, but how can I be certain that my symptoms do not indicate bowel cancer or any other potentially dangerous disease?*

A A GP will be able to confirm the diagnosis of IBS from the symptoms you describe (see earlier question). A general examination, even with particular attention to the abdomen, will not yield any particular signs of IBS. Further tests are usually unnecessary, although blood tests are often done to check that the liver is functioning properly, and for anaemia, which may be a sign of bowel cancer (see later in this chapter). If there is any doubt about the diagnosis, examination of the lower end of the bowel by a telescope put into the back passage (sigmoidoscopy) may be recommended. This will involve referral to a surgeon. People who are over 45 when the symptoms start, and who have a family history of bowel cancer, may be referred to a physician for an examination of all of the lower bowel (colonoscopy), as well as a sigmoidoscopy.

Itchy bottom

Common causes of an itchy bottom	
Threadworm	Allergic reactions
Piles	Thrush (see Chapters 4 and 5)

Threadworm

Q *I have an itch in and around my back passage that is driving me demented. It keeps me awake at night, and I often find I am surreptitiously scratching myself in the middle of the day. My kids are scratching their bottoms too. Do you have any advice?*

A One of the most common causes of itchy bottoms is threadworm, and given that you have children in the house who are also scratching, this is the most likely cause of your torment.

Threadworms are elusive little creatures, which you may never spot. They are transmitted by bad hygiene – which can easily happen with little children. For example, a small child with threadworm may get tiny bits of poo on his or her hands and transfer it to toys, playmates, siblings or you. These people then put their own hands in their mouths, and so the threadworm enters their guts and emerges from their bottoms a couple of weeks later. Scrupulous hand-washing after going to the toilet or using the potty is ideal, but not always possible.

The most effective treatment is to treat the whole family with a single dose of mebendazole (Vermox), available over the counter and suitable for everyone except children under two and pregnant women. A follow-up dose two weeks later could help prevent re-infection.

Remind the whole family that everyone must wash their hands and scrub their nails after each visit to the toilet and before meals. Keeping nails short is a sensible precaution. Tell staff at your children's school about the infection, so they can reinforce the hygiene message.

Piles

Q *I am sometimes plagued by a very itchy back passage and I have noticed a bit of blood on the toilet paper when I wipe myself. I think I have got piles. What should I do?*

A Piles (also known as haemorrhoids) are amazingly common. They are like varicose veins of the back passage, where different vein systems come together and can become twisted and engorged. Constipation and straining to pass stools may irritate the piles, causing bright-red bleeding which you will see on the toilet paper when you wipe yourself, itchiness and a lump which sticks out of your back passage after straining but which can usually be pushed back in with your finger. Soothing creams available over the counter, such as Anusol or Germoloids, may help the itch. Suppositories containing steroids, anaesthetic and soothing agents, such as Xyloproct or Anusol-HC, are available only on prescription but tend to be more effective than cream alone.

However, if you have weight loss, unexplained bleeding from your back passage or changes in your bowel habits, you need to see a doctor, because it could be a sign of bowel cancer (see below).

Allergies

Q *My bottom has become very itchy but my GP assures me I do not have piles. I took treatment for threadworm, but that has not helped, and no one else in the family is scratching. What else could the cause of the itchiness be?*

A An itchy bottom could be caused by an allergy – usually to soap, bubble baths, perfumes or soap powders. If you find that the itch starts after you have started using a new soap or detergent, stop using the product immediately. (Otherwise, try a process of elimination to discover what is causing the allergic reaction.) You could take an oral antihistamine (e.g. Clarityn, Hismanal or Piriton), available over the counter, to ease the itch.

Bleeding from the back passage

Possible causes of bleeding from the back passage

Piles

Diverticulitis (see below)

Gut diseases, e.g. **Crohn's disease** (see page 198)

Q *I have had some bright-red blood on the toilet paper when I wipe myself after opening my bowels. Could it be serious?*

A Piles (see above) are the most common cause of bright-red bleeding from the back passage.

A more unusual cause is diverticulitis, which is an inflammation of small pouches (diverticulae) that develop in the wall of the large bowel, usually in the last section that passes down the left side of your abdomen. Bits of faeces can get stuck in these pouches, causing the inflammation, which you experience as a sudden onset of pain and tenderness on the lower left side of the abdomen, in addition to passing bright-red blood. You may also feel feverish and unwell.

Go to your GP if you have these symptoms: these flare-ups are usually treated with strong antibiotics and painkillers. You can help yourself by taking measures such as eating a medium-fibre diet, drinking plenty of fluids and exercising to keep the stool flowing smoothly. You could also try anti-spasmodic drugs, e.g. mebeverine (Colofac) to alleviate gripey pain; peppermints if you feel bloated; and anti-diarrhoeal drugs, e.g. loperamide (Imodium, Arret, Diocalm Ultra) to stop the diarrhoea if the stool gets too loose. Above all, see your GP if you get any bleeding from the back passage or the pattern of your stool changes, as you must not assume that all bowel problems are necessarily to do with piles or diverticulitis.

Q *How do I know whether the bleeding I occasionally get from my back passage is caused by piles or heralds the beginning of bowel cancer?*

A Serious underlying bowel diseases, such as Crohn's disease and ulcerative colitis (see pages 198–9), which cause inflammation of the bowel, and bowel cancer, are rarer than piles and diverticulitis. However, it is always wise to get any bleeding from the back passage or other unexplained bowel problems checked by your GP and to request a referral to a specialist if any doubt remains.

Spots around the back passage

Q *I am a gay man and I have anal warts. I have had them before and had to attend a clinic on several occasions to have the warts frozen off. My partner has not got any, and has accused me of sleeping around, which I have not done. I am mortified to have warts again and cannot face going to the clinic. What should I do?*

A Most people who have anal, or genital, warts find that they disappear within six months whether they have been treated or not. But up to 30 per cent of infected people find that the warts persist or else clear up and then recur months or even years later. So you can tell your partner that it does not mean you have been sleeping around. In fact, he may be the source of your warts himself because some people infected with the wart virus (human papilloma virus) never develop visible warts. The good news for you is that there has been a move away from clinic treatments towards giving people the medication to use in their own homes. Two creams are used commonly: podophyllotoxin (Warticon) and imiquimod (Aldara). The former works quickly and is cheap, the latter takes longer but gives a more lasting result with fewer relapses. However, not everyone likes treating themselves – this is something to discuss at the clinic, which you should attend.

(See Chapter 3 for more about genital warts and other sexually transmitted diseases.)

Bowel cancer

Bowel cancers are known as colorectal cancers. They are the second most common cause of death from cancer in the UK, after lung cancer, accounting for 20,000 deaths a year. They are rare in people under 40 and are usually found in people who are in their fifties, sixties or older.

There is no single cause of bowel cancer. However, a diet high in animal fats and food preservatives, and low in fibre, may put you at increased risk, and there is some evidence that taking calcium and selenium may help to protect against bowel disease. There may also be an inherited tendency to bowel cancer.

The most common symptoms are change of bowel habit and rectal bleeding, although these are also very common in people who do not have cancer. (Nearly 20 per cent of us have bleeding from the bottom every year and a third of us suffer from constipation.) It is therefore important to know the higher-risk symptoms and to act on them.

The changes in **bowel habit** you should act on are recent, persistent changes that last for a few weeks without returning to normal. These include a change to looser, more diarrhoea-like motions, or to going to the toilet (or trying to go) several more times a day than normal. The symptoms are especially significant if accompanied by bleeding.

The changes in **rectal bleeding** you should act on are those which happen persistently, without any apparent reason. Piles are the main cause of rectal bleeding but piles usually have other symptoms such as straining, sore bottom, lumps and itching. In older people (e.g. over 60), rectal bleeding should always be investigated because piles could

---

Slime or mucus from the back passage

Possible causes of slime or mucus when you open your bowels

Irritable bowel syndrome (IBS) (See above)

Piles (See above)

Crohn's disease or **ulcerative colitis** (See above)

be masking more serious symptoms. Other higher-risk symptoms in this age group include:

- unexplained anaemia found by your GP
- a lump or mass in your tummy felt by your GP
- persistent, colicky, severe abdominal pain, which has come on recently for the first time.

Most people with these higher-risk symptoms do not have cancer, but if you have any of these you should get advice from your GP and be referred for hospital investigation if the symptoms have persisted for a few weeks.

Investigations for suspected bowel cancer include a blood test to check for anaemia, checking stool samples for traces of blood, and a rectal examination. A specialist at the hospital may give you a sigmoidoscopy and/or a colonoscopy. Barium enemas may also be advised, and there may be further tests.

The treatment also depends on the type and position of the cancer. All will involve an operation. The most common type and site of rectal cancers allow the segment of bowel containing the cancer to be cut out and the ends of bowel sewn back together, avoiding the need for a colostomy. Most people make a quick and full recovery from surgery.

Chemotherapy is sometimes advised to mop up any possible cancer cells that may remain. Bowel cancers that have not spread and are confined to that section of the bowel have an excellent outlook after surgery, with 80 per cent of people surviving more than five years, after which recurrence becomes unlikely.

(See Chapter 1 for more about cancer.)

Q *I have noticed that there is some jelly-like slime when I wipe myself after opening my bowels and sometimes on top of the stool itself. Should I be concerned?*

A Slime or mucus implies that there is inflammation or irritation in part of the gut. It often accompanies piles or can be a sign of IBS or, less often, a sign of an inflammatory bowel disease such as Crohn's or ulcerative colitis. If it happens more than once, or is accompanied by other symptoms – such as bleeding, abdominal pain, constipation or diarrhoea, stools that float on the surface of the water in the toilet and don't flush away, or weight loss – then it is more likely to be a sign of underlying disease such as Crohn's, and you need to see a doctor within a few days. If there are none of those symptoms, it is most likely to be a sign of IBS. (See earlier in this chapter for more about this.)

Faecal incontinence

Q *I have a horribly embarrassing problem. I find that I stain my knickers most days. Sometimes there are even small lumps of faeces in them and I am terrified that I will start to smell. I am very reluctant to go to a gym, swimming pool or beach because I would find it so awful if anyone were to see my stained clothing. There does not seem to be anything wrong with my bowels although I do get constipated sometimes. Can you help?*

A Faecal incontinence or soiling can often be easily treated and the first step is to overcome your embarrassment and head for your GP. It affects up to one in twenty people and is caused by a malfunction of either the bowel or the muscular ring (sphincter) around the back passage, which allows stool, liquid or gas to escape when you do not want it to.

Faecal incontinence can affect any age group, and the causes depend on the age of the person affected:

- **children and teenagers** – if they are born with an abnormal sphincter or if they have persistent constipation (which means that loose bits of stool can leak around the constipation and dribble out of the anus)
- **women following childbirth** – owing to a hidden or obvious tear in the sphincter muscles

- **elderly people** – because of constipation and overflow from the bowel owing to failing mental capacity or to sphincter damage persisting from a younger age.

People of any age who experience an injury or infection of the sphincter may be affected immediately or in later life. Those suffering from inflammatory bowel disease (such as Crohn's disease or ulcerative colitis) or IBS (which can cause alternating constipation and diarrhoea, together with abdominal pain) are at risk because the bowel is very sensitive. Disorders such as multiple sclerosis, stroke and epilepsy can result in damage to the nerves supplying the sphincter, so people who suffer from them could have faecal incontinence too.

To find out the cause of your incontinence, you may need tests to measure your sphincter function, including an ultrasound scan of the sphincter muscle itself. Treatment will depend on the underlying cause.

People with faecal incontinence quickly learn to identify and stay away from foods or situations that make them more likely to leak faeces in public. Most will leave plenty of time to empty their bowels before going out, will take a drug to prevent diarrhoea, such as loperamide (Imodium, Arret, Diocalm Ultra), if that helps them not to pass faeces, and will always carry a change of underwear, scented nappy bags to carry soiled clothes, wear pads inside pants and carry a deodorising spray.

However, no one should have to live with faecal incontinence. It is important to seek medical help and if you are not satisfied, be referred to a specialist centre with a team which runs a service geared to helping those with your problem. Support is available from the Continence Foundation,★ which has a helpline, and Incontact.★

Chapter 8

Personal hygiene

Most of us feel self-conscious, from time to time, about our bodily smells. The human body is a complex organism with a sophisticated mechanism for keeping itself clean and healthy. Sweating, for example, performs the essential functions of cooling down the body and getting rid of some waste chemicals. The irony is that in our modern society, where people live in close confinement and spend long periods of time indoors, the products of our body's self-cleaning system can smell.

Some degree of smell is natural and attractive and, as long as we wash sufficiently often and thoroughly, should not cause offence. Indeed, an antipathy to natural body odours may lead to excessive use of perfumed products, which can themselves be overpowering to other people. There is also a risk of allergies arising from overuse of potentially toxic chemicals on the skin.

Certain parts of the body do generate potentially smelly waste products, however – and sweaty armpits, smelly feet, vaginal smells and bad breath can be a problem. Such embarrassing smells can cause distress and anxiety about the possible effect on your social life or even job prospects.

This chapter looks at the possible causes of unpleasant odours from these parts of the body, suggests what you can do to combat them yourself, and describes the medical options that are available if necessary. Details of support organisations are given at the back of the book.

Glossary

Gingivitis Gum disease

Halitosis Bad breath

Hyperhidrosis Excessive sweating

Plaque Build-up of bacteria between teeth and between gums and teeth

Sympathectomy An operation to destroy the sympathetic nerves, which control sweating

Bad breath

Most of us have temporary bad breath at times, particularly first thing in the morning. Plaque or food residues can build up overnight, and the smell of strong foods, alcohol or cigarettes consumed the previous night often lingers. Our saliva helps to keep the mouth clean, and we produce less of this at night.

More persistent bad breath may have a number of causes. If plaque is allowed to build up it can result in gingivitis (gum disease). Occasionally halitosis may be a side-effect of medication, and, very rarely, it might be an indication of internal disease.

Further advice about bad breath is available from various organisations and web sites. These include the Fresh Breath Centre,★ the London Breath Centre★ and Bad Breath Research.★

Common causes of temporary halitosis
Dry mouth first thing in the morning
Certain foods and chemicals
Smoking
Alcohol

Possible causes of long-lasting halitosis
Plaque
Gingivitis or **acute necrotising ulcerative gingivitis (ANUG)**
Certain drugs
Internal disease (rarely)

Temporary bad breath

Q *My breath is really stale in the mornings and I sometimes feel it is a bit 'off' during the day. At other times, I feel my breath is fresh as a daisy. Why should this be so?*

A Stale breath in the mornings usually reflects what you have eaten the night before. Large chunks of garlic, pickles and spices stay on the breath, as does alcohol. Smoking cigars, pipes and cigarettes can also make the breath stale and leave a lingering odour because smoke dries out the mouth and there is less saliva to rinse away the smell (see Chapter 1 for advice on quitting smoking). Even if you do not eat smelly foods, smoke or drink alcohol, your breath may be stale in the mornings because bacteria work overnight on any small residues of food in the mouth, so make sure that you brush your teeth well before going to bed. Snorers, who tend to sleep with their mouths open, are prone to having dry mouths, so their breath may be smellier than that of non-snorers in the morning.

Q *What can I do about my bad breath? I've tried lots of different mouthwashes and sprays but the smell seems to keep coming through.*

A First, check whether you really do have bad breath – ask either a good friend or your dentist. Check your gums and if they bleed easily on contact or look inflamed book an appointment with the dental hygienist for a scale and polish. Six-monthly dental check-ups are a good way to prevent gum disease (see below).

Pay close attention to daily flossing, twice-daily brushing, and avoiding foods that linger on the breath. Mouthwashes are no substitute for good cleaning and there is a small risk that by using them you will be getting rid of 'good' bacteria too, that help digest food and keep the mouth free of fungal infections.

Electric toothbrushes tend to clean better than manual ones but it depends on how you use them – a thorough clean with a manual one is still better than a hurried scrub with an electric brush.

Sugar-free chewing gum and drinks of water and lemon help to freshen the breath.

Gingivitis

Q *I have had bad breath for some time now and it doesn't seem to be getting any better. I have also noticed that my gums bleed and look swollen. What could be causing it and what can I do to clear it up?*

A Some persistent halitosis can be a result of gingivitis, a gum infection. If your gums bleed when you brush them and the gum looks swollen where it meets the tooth, it is very likely that you have gingivitis. The inflammation of the gums is caused by a build-up of plaque, which is an accumulation of bacteria between the teeth and where the teeth meet the gum. The waste products of the bacterial action (from both the plaque itself and the gingivitis) on food debris cause a foul, stale smell. If the gingivitis is not treated, in time your teeth would become loose and fall out.

If you have long-term halitosis it could be a result of acute necrotising ulcerative gingivitis (ANUG), which is a severe form of gingivitis and is also known as trench mouth or Vincent's angina. Treatment involves antibiotics and serious descaling work by a dentist.

Medication

Q *I am taking lots of tablets for various ailments. A friend said this mixture could be causing my bad breath. Is this possible?*

A Drugs that dry out the mouth can cause bad breath: prime examples are antidepressants such as amitriptyline (Lentizol), hyoscine (Buscopan), which is used for irritable bowel syndrome, and anti-incontinence drugs such as oxybutynin (Ditropan).

Talk to your GP about which of your tablets could be causing your dry mouth and whether you can change or come off them.

Internal disease

Q *I have been told that my bad breath could mean there's something wrong with me inside. Is this an old wives' tale?*

A On the whole, bad breath reflects your dental hygiene. However, in certain cases it can be an indication of an internal disease. For example, a characteristic sweet smell can denote the presence of ketones, which can occur when you are very hungry (or if you are denying yourself food because you are anorexic) or by diabetics whose blood sugar levels are uncontrolled. It is often said that gut problems such as constipation can cause bad breath, but experts dispute this.

Breath analysis, in which a test analyses a chemical constituent of your breath to check for a specific condition, is currently used in diagnosing the bacterial infection *Helicobacter pylori*, which is associated with stomach ulcers.

Vaginal smells

Normal vaginas are not odourless. Some vaginal discharge is natural and helps to keep the vagina clean. You may be more aware of a smell when your hormones alter, such as before a period, when pregnant or when you start the contraceptive pill. A smell of stale blood may be noticeable if you use sanitary towels during a period. Many women notice a distinctive smell from the vagina in the morning if they have had sex the night before.

There are various possible causes of an abnormal, persistent vaginal smell, the commonest being the infection bacterial vaginosis (BV). Another infection, trichomonas, also generates a smelly discharge – as does a tampon, eventually, if you forget to remove it.

Further advice is available from the organisation Women's Health.*

Possible causes of vaginal smells

Poor hygiene	Trichomonas
Bacterial vaginosis (BV)	Forgotten tampon

Hygiene

Q *I feel that my vagina sometimes smells, but I have had every test under the sun and they have all been negative. Is there any vaginal deodorant I could use?*

A Vaginal deodorants are not generally a good idea as they may cause irritation and destroy useful bacteria that help keep thrush at bay (see Chapter 5). They may also cause allergic reactions that result in itching and soreness. It is far better to establish a regular routine of personal hygiene. This involves washing your genitals daily, drying them properly and wearing clean, preferably cotton, knickers every day. Try to avoid synthetic leggings or tights as these tend to trap sweat, which causes a smell as it is broken down by bacteria.

Bacterial vaginosis

Q *I had a test at my GP's because of a smelly vaginal discharge and was told I had bacterial vaginosis. What is this and what can I do about it?*

A Bacterial vaginosis (BV) is also known as anaerobic vaginosis. The smell, which is fishy, is often more pronounced after sexual intercourse. There will usually be a discharge from the vagina as well as the fishy smell. The discharge is watery and a greyish, off-white colour. It does not cause soreness or irritation.

You cannot catch BV from a sexual partner; it is caused by an over-growth of bacteria – mainly gardnerella – which are normally present in the vagina. The reason why this imbalance occurs is unclear.

In the past, bacterial vaginosis was thought to be harmless. However, it may increase the risk of pelvic inflammatory disease (PID), which is an infection of the Fallopian tubes (see Chapter 5).

Treatment for BV is a course of oral antibiotics (usually metronidazole). There is now evidence that BV doubles the likelihood of preterm labour (going into labour after 24 weeks of pregnancy but before the baby is due), so if you are intending to become pregnant you should have the condition treated beforehand, as metronidazole should not be taken during pregnancy.

(See Chapter 5 for more about BV.)

Trichomonas

Q *I have a greenish discharge from my vagina that does not smell nice. It looks a bit bubbly. Do I need to get it checked?*

A You might have an infection known as trichomonas. This is caused by a tiny amoeba-like (protozoan) organism called *Trichomonas vaginalis*. It causes a discharge that is often frothy and yellowish-green, but which may also be thin and scanty. The discharge is smelly, and the vulva is often sore. It may also be painful to pass urine.

Trichomonas is a sexually transmitted disease, but male partners may be unaware of their condition as most men with trichomonas do not have any symptoms. It is not dangerous, although some doctors think it could possibly spread to the Fallopian tubes.

You need to see your GP or attend a family planning clinic or a sexually transmitted diseases clinic for checks and advice. The treatment is usually a course of oral antibiotics. A swab (cotton bud on a long stick) can be taken from any vaginal discharge to make a firm diagnosis.

Gonorrhoea is a rarer cause of smelly discharge and the swabs will test for gonorrhoea also.

As both trichomonas and gonorrhoea are sexually transmitted, your partner will need to be screened too. (See Chapter 3 for more about sexually transmitted diseases.)

Forgotten tampon

Q *I have noticed a nasty smell from my vagina that has been getting worse since my last period. In the past few days I've noticed a greenish, thick discharge which stinks. What could it be?*

A A forgotten tampon is a common cause of vaginal discharge. After a week or two the tampon begins to fester, and there will be a foul-smelling discharge. If you suspect you may have forgotten to remove your last tampon, you need to see your GP.

It is particularly important to remove tampons every eight hours and not to leave them in for longer, if possible, in order to avoid the risk of toxic shock syndrome. This is a rare but potentially fatal infection caused by a toxin (poison), produced by a bacterium called *Staphylococcus aureus*. It can produce collapse, confusion, fever, a rash, diarrhoea, and muscle pains. Hospital admission is necessary and intravenous fluids and antibiotics are administered.

Smelly feet

Smelly feet are sweaty feet. The average man loses half a pint of sweat a day through his feet. The sweat itself does not smell but bacteria break it down into fatty acids, which have the characteristic acrid smell.

The answer is to keep the feet dry and clean. Synthetic socks and tights (i.e. those that are not made from natural fibres, such as cotton or silk) or shoes with linings that do not let the feet breathe, help to keep the feet moist with sweat and keep the smells ripe and putrid.

Special treatments are available for those who have a severe problem with excessive sweating of the feet.

Infections of the feet are a rarer cause of smells, but the fungal infection athlete's foot and a condition called keratolysis are both possible culprits.

Athlete's foot makes the skin between the toes red, soggy and usually very itchy. The nails may look discoloured and misshapen too. Antifungal creams, powders or oral tablets are the best treatment.

Keratolysis causes small pits in the soles of the feet and is due to a particular bacterium which gains hold after you have worn boots for long periods of time, especially in humid conditions. Antibiotics are usually necessary to clear it up.

Further advice is available from the web site of the Society of Chiropodists and Podiatrists.★

Common causes of smelly feet

Sweat   This may be exacerbated by synthetic socks or shoe linings

Fungal infection   (e.g. athlete's foot)

Bacterial infection   (e.g. keratolysis)

Q *What can I do about my smelly, sweaty feet? All my trainers stink and I have to throw them out after a few months. My friends are always moaning about my smelly feet and I'm embarrassed to take my shoes off. Do you have any advice?*

A Keeping your feet clean and dry will go some way to helping with the smell. Wash your feet daily in warm water. Try adding a few drops of tea tree oil to the water (this is an antiseptic, which keeps the feet clear of foul-smelling bacteria). Dry your feet thoroughly – between the toes and round the nail bed. Wear socks that have a high cotton content (but not pure cotton). Wash them well, with dilute antiseptic, if necessary. Change your shoes regularly and do not wear trainers for too long at a time.

A foot antiperspirant/deodorant is no substitute for washing. However, if you do use one it should contain 20 per cent aluminium chloride solution (e.g. Perspirex, Driclor, Anhydrol Forte – available from pharmacies). Use at night after washing the feet thoroughly. However, do not use if you have a fungal infection or open cracks on your feet.

If the problem persists, consult your GP.

Q *I have tried every spray, powder and product available in the chemist's for smelly feet. I have a real problem in that my feet get so sweaty that they slide around inside my shoes, and the smell is impossible to control. Is there any further help available?*

A Desperate problems call for desperate solutions. Your GP can refer you for any of the following treatments as you obviously have a severe problem.

If you have seriously sweaty feet, you may want to consider botulinum toxin injections. This inactivates the nerves that trigger sweat-gland activity. The treatment is tedious and uncomfortable because you may need over 30 of the tiny injections into the soles of your feet, and the skin of the feet is very sensitive. This is a new treatment so it may not be available in your local hospital, but your GP can find out the location of the nearest specialist treatment centre.

Anticholinergic drugs (drugs that reduce sweating), such as propantheline bromide, can be prescribed by your GP. These block the action of the nerves responsible for sweating, and are therefore fairly effective. However, their side-effects – drying of the mouth, blurring of vision, constipation and sedation – may be worse than the sweating.

A technique called iontophoresis available in some private centres and a few NHS hospital departments may help. An electric current is passed through a liquid containing an anticholinergic drug directly on to the sole of the foot. The idea is that the drug penetrates the sole of the foot to reduce sweating. You need to have weekly sessions at first, then every month. The treatment does not hurt and works well for some people, though evidence for its effectiveness is limited.

A sympathectomy operation (see page 219) to destroy the nerves that control sweating of the feet is possible, but only in the most severe cases.

Body odour

Body odour (BO) is, like smelly feet, caused by bacterial break-down of sweat. Fresh sweat does not normally produce an unpleasant odour; it is stale sweat that smells, because bacteria that live on the surface of the skin break the sweat down, releasing certain pungent chemicals. Areas of the body such as the armpits produce a special type of sweat that is more likely to go stale because it contains fats and proteins that encourage bacteria to grow, whereas the sweat from other parts of the body is mainly salt water.

As with smelly feet, the remedy for body odour is regular and thorough washing, drying properly and avoiding clothes made from synthetic fibres, which trap sweat. You can also use chemicals such as antiperspirants to prevent sweat or mask its effects. New deodorants that break down sweat into carbon dioxide rather than the usual smelly fatty acids are being developed. As with smelly feet, special treatments, including surgery, are possible for extreme cases of excessive sweating.

Q *A close friend told me the other day that I have BO and need to do something about it, as other friends have commented on it to her. Naturally I was mortified and deeply upset. What can I do about it?*

A You could take a number of measures if you think – or are told – you have BO. As a first step, check if you really do by asking another close friend to confirm, and by sniffing your clothes at the end of the day to see if they smell stale.

If you want to do away with the problem, try the following:

- wash more often, especially when it is hot – you may need to shower twice a day in the summer
- use a deodorant or an antiperspirant – the former masks smells and the latter stops you sweating
- use a stronger antiperspirant (e.g. Drichlor) if regular ones are not enough and apply it at night
- wash your clothes at the end of every day and wear a fresh T-shirt or top and underwear every day.

Q *I seem to sweat extremely heavily both during the day and at night. I take in a clean shirt to work and have to change at lunchtime as the one I put on* *in the morning is stained and damp by midday. My forehead runs with sweat and I am finding it more and more difficult to function in the office and have a social life. I shower every morning, wear a fresh shirt and underwear every day, have tried antiperspirants, talc – you name it, I've tried it. I am at my wits' end. What can I do?*

A It is obviously uncomfortable and embarrassing to sweat as much as you do. You should first take time to find out why you are sweating so much before embarking on expensive and invasive treatments. The possible causes are:

- **anxiety** (see Chapter 2)
- **hot or poorly ventilated rooms** Others in your workplace may also be finding the office too hot but may be keeping it to themselves. Ask your colleagues and speak to management about better air conditioning or ventilation if you all feel the same way
- **a high metabolic rate** If you have an overactive thyroid, your metabolic rate will be high. Sweats, tremor, weight loss and palpitations are other possible symptoms. A blood test can determine whether your thyroid is normal
- **fevers or ill health** If you are drenched in sweat and are feeling unwell, perhaps excessively tired, it is worth having a blood test to check your full blood count which can indicate underlying infection and blood diseases. An examination by your GP to check that you have no enlarged glands (lymph nodes) is also a good idea. If you have returned from a holiday to a tropical area and are having recurrent fevers and sweats, you need a blood test for malaria
- **hyperhidrosis** Some people just sweat more than others for no apparent cause. Attending to personal hygiene as you are doing is the best way of managing it. You will also want to avoid things that make you pour with sweat (e.g. hot, stuffy restaurants, spicy foods and alcohol). Wear light-coloured, non-synthetic, loose clothing rather than dark, tight synthetics.

Some specialised treatments are available, mainly in the private sector. Botulinum toxin, a poison, can be injected into the skin to render inactive the nerves that stimulate the sweat glands so they do not produce as much sweat. One treatment session of ten injections into your armpit should reduce sweating for at least six months (the effect will not last forever). A more major operation to control sweating is called a **sympathectomy**. Under general anaesthetic, the nerves that control sweating (sympathetic nervous system), which run through your chest wall, are destroyed. The operation works in about a third of cases but the main drawback is that you may notice increased sweating in other parts of your body, usually on your chest and back and sometimes on your feet. To have a major operation and then find that you have sweaty feet rather than sweaty armpits is a bit of a blow to say the least, and the operation is irreversible so you are stuck with the results.

Chapter 9

Skin, hair and nails

The way many of us treat our skin, hair and nails, it is not surprising that they sometimes cause us problems. The sun and the numerous chemicals and pollutants to which they are exposed would destroy most other materials. For the most part, they serve us well; but because they are so visible to other people, it can cause a great deal of embarrassment and humiliation when unpleasant conditions do occur.

Few people escape their fair share of spots in adolescence, but for some these continue into adulthood, and if you suffer from severe acne the problem may seem to take over your life. Rashes can cause misery, particularly if they are very itchy and you have to keep scratching in public. Fungal and parasitic infections, such as scabies, can be mortifying, especially as there is some stigma attached to them, which might make you reluctant to go to the doctor.

Our skin deteriorates as we age; many people suffer from thread veins and varicose veins, and no one escapes wrinkles. Those who have spent holidays in the sun for years know that the flip-side of sunbathing is the risk of skin cancer – and we worry about changes in our moles and the significance of any lumps or bumps.

Hair and nail problems, too, may be caused by the damage we do to them – hair that falls out because of years of bleaching, or nails that become flaky because of repeated washing-up without gloves. As with skin conditions, the cosmetic effect of thinning hair, hair growing where you don't want it to, or discoloured or infected nails can be very upsetting. These symptoms could also be a sign of an underlying medical condition.

This chapter gives advice about the possible causes of all these problems, in addition to others, such as dandruff. (For head lice, see Chapter 11.) It offers guidance about treatment options, including self-help for chronic conditions, such as eczema and psoriasis, which tend to recur, and do not have a cure. However, a judicious use of conventional and complementary therapies can ease symptoms and help to control the problem, and contact with self-help groups can provide good information and support. Details of such groups are given at the back of the book.

Glossary

Acne   Skin condition resulting in blackheads, cysts, spots. Common in adolescence; possible at any age

Alopecia   Hair loss

Antihistamine   A drug that blocks the effects of histamine, which is produced in the body in response to injury or damage, and causes itching

Collagen   The cement between cells that binds tissues together

Dermatologist   Skin specialist

Eczema   Long-term skin condition causing dry, irritated skin

Epidermis   Outermost layer of skin

Intertrigo   Soreness in skin creases, e.g. under breasts or in the groin. Often caused by fungal infections such as thrush

Macule   A different-coloured patch of skin (e.g. pale on dark-skinned people; brown or red on light-skinned people)

Melanin   Pigment that gives skin its colour

Melanoma   Malignant growth of cells containing melanin

Psoriasis   Long-term skin condition causing dry, scaly patches on the elbows, knees and scalp, and sometimes pitted nails and painful joints

---

Skin

Skin conditions may be alarming, upsetting and embarrassing, but they are very rarely life-threatening. Even the majority of skin cancers are treatable, although malignant melanoma can be fatal. Lumps and bumps should always be checked out if they persist for more than a couple of weeks or are accompanied by other symptoms. Moles should be monitored carefully too if they begin to change shape and colour.

The skin can be a very useful indicator of internal disease. Many conditions such as diabetes, joint complaints (e.g. lupus and rheumatoid arthritis), heart diseases and infectious diseases such as meningitis, cause rashes that are characteristic and aid diagnosis – so if you develop any worrying skin problem, see your doctor.

Itchy or scaly rashes, blisters

Possible causes of rashes

Eczema

Psoriasis

Fungal infections   (e.g. intertrigo, ringworm)

Seborrhoeic dermatitis

Scabies

Possible causes of blisters

Burns

Insect bites

Chickenpox

Shingles   Reactivation of chickenpox virus (e.g. because you are run down or for no known reason) that you had earlier in your life. Not due to recent contact with chickenpox

Herpes (cold sores)   (See Chapter 10)

Allergic reaction   (e.g. to drugs, foods or chemicals)

Itchy rash

Q *I get patches of eczema which flare up when I am stressed or eat strawberries and in the hayfever season. I am not that bothered by its appearance – it is not very visible – but the itchiness drives me demented. I have tried strong steroid creams, such as Betnovate, for years but have been warned by my GP not to keep using it because it thins the skin. I have also noticed that it is much less effective when I use it a lot. What else can I do?*

A In the case of eczema, prevention is the best option, although it is admittedly hard in your case, especially if it means staying indoors during the hayfever season (usually March to September, but depends on the weather, which pollens you are sensitive to, etc.) Moisturising your skin with a bath oil, soap substitute or a cream such as aqueous cream or E45 can keep the eczema in check. Oral antihistamines, such as Clarityn (which does not make you tired), or Piriton (which does), can relieve the itch. A new cream called doxepin 5 per cent cream (Xepin-Bioglan), which is an antidepressant drug made into a cream, is being marketed specifically to relieve the itch of eczema. It may make you tired. However, a recent review by Consumers' Association's *Drug and Therapeutics Bulletin* said that, based on current evidence, doxepin cream cannot be recommended.

Acupuncture and homeopathy help some sufferers from eczema. Chinese herbal remedies are popular too, but you do not necessarily know what you are swallowing until all herbalists agree to have their remedies standardised and tested.

Q *Very unusually, I am always relieved when the summer is over. This is because embarrassing and unsightly bumps at the tops of my arms mean I cannot wear sleeveless tops. I am quite fair-skinned and the bumps look alarmingly obvious. Is there anything I can do before next summer so that I don't have to keep my arms under wraps again?*

A You do not have to have perfect arms in order to enjoy wearing a sleeveless top in the summer. It is hard to find a woman who thinks her upper arms or thighs are faultless, but most of us show off our less-than-perfect limbs regardless. You probably have a very common skin condition called keratosis pilaris, which tends to run in families. There is no cure for it and it does not have any sinister implications – it is really just a cosmetic problem. It causes tiny rough spots on the outer part of the arms and occasionally the thighs. It affects teenagers mainly and tends to become less obvious as you get older. The spots may look red and rough but rarely itch and never hurt or become cancerous. The condition occurs because as the skin renews itself old skin cells get stuck in the hair follicles and make a scaly plug of dead cells. Try using a moisturising cream (e.g. Diprobase) twice a day, rub your arms with a pumice stone or loofah when showering or bathing, and consider getting a prescription for tretinoin (Retin-A) cream or gel. For the first few weeks of treatment, Retin A may cause redness and peeling of the skin but after that the bumps may flatten out nicely.

Q *I am a 40-year-old man and have been suffering from an infuriating itching on my legs for the last year or so. It is especially prevalent when I get out of the bath or expose my legs to the air. The only visible sign is that my legs go a bit red and blotchy at the time, which is not helped by scratching. I have tried aloe vera gel and other creams, but they have a very short-term effect. Odd as it sounds, the only thing that has given me any relief is when my legs had to be shaved for an operation. I had no itching at all, until the hair grew back after a couple of weeks. I am at my wits' end – what else can I do?*

A It sounds as though you may have a form of eczema which is dry, irritated, itchy skin; although it is hard to be certain. As it just seems to affect your legs it could be something external that is often in contact with your skin. For example, do you play golf in knee-length trousers? Do you garden wearing clothes that would allow grass etc. to come into contact with your legs and irritate them? Do you have a cat that rubs against your legs? Do you wear long socks that could be irritating your skin, and so on?

If you can identify potential triggers, you can try avoiding or eliminating them. Failing that, you could try to treat the symptoms with:

- an oral antihistamine tablet (e.g. Piriton), at night to reduce scratching
- a heavy-duty moisturiser twice a day and after bathing (e.g. Neutrogena dermatological cream) or even Vaseline
- a bath oil such as Oilatum.

Avoid soaps, aloe vera, and other creams for the time being. If there is no improvement, see your GP and ask to be referred to a dermatologist. The National Eczema Society* can also supply useful advice.

Q *I have had an itching in my pubic hair area and the creases of my groin for several months now. I also have a small patch underneath one breast. It itches like mad and I am making my skin bleed with scratching. What is wrong and what should I use to soothe it?*

A It may be a fungal infection. An antifungal cream such as clotrimazole (Canesten) might help. Fungi thrive in hot, moist places, so skin creases and crevices, such as the skin under the breasts, are favourite breeding grounds. This kind of irritated skin, often caused by a fungal infection, is called intertrigo and is particularly common if you have diabetes. Red, slightly itchy, scaly patches can also occur as a form of psoriasis, in which the skin becomes heaped up into bumps – although you would usually have a scaly scalp and patches elsewhere on the body too. Eczema is the other common cause of itchy patches on the skin, but does not usually occur just in skin creases.

Try using the Canesten cream at least three times a day for seven days, keeping the skin very dry and sweat-free. If it is fungal intertrigo, it should clear up. If it does not, ask your GP to have a look – a few days of a steroid cream will clear it up if it is psoriasis or eczema in most cases (although this will make it worse if it is fungal). However, it may then recur when you stop the cream.

Q *I have developed a sore red rash on my face, which itches occasionally. I have tried a mild steroid cream (hydrocortisone) and this has had no effect. When I first get up in the morning it seems quite calm, but gets worse as the day goes on. I have not changed my make-up or soap or washing products. Should I change them, and what else can I do?*

A Your itchy rash could be:

- **eczema** This causes dry, itchy skin. It is sometimes triggered by an allergy (e.g. to soap or face cream). Try not using soap or chemicals on your face, including make-up. Instead use a light moisturising cream, such as aqueous cream, and take an antihistamine tablet (e.g. Piriton) at night to soothe the itch and irritation. If the rash persists, see your doctor
- **acne** If you have blackheads and pimples, you may have developed acne. It can come on at any age and may be related to your hormones. Some drugs such as steroids can cause acne. It is prudent to ask your GP to confirm this diagnosis because anti-acne creams such as benzoyl peroxide (Panoxyl), can make eczema worse
- **rosacea** A red face with pimples and broken blood vessels on the cheeks and nose, which gets worse when you drink alcohol, may be rosacea (see also pages 229 and 239). See your GP for diagnosis
- **seborrhoeic dermatitis** This is a long-term condition which, like eczema and psoriasis, cannot be cured but does wax and

wane. It causes severe dandruff and scaling of the eyebrows, which can inflame your eyelids and irritate your eyes. You can also develop scaling in the middle of the face, back, breastbone, armpits and groin. Steroid creams can give relief in the short term, but should not be used long-term. Creams that reduce the scaling may also be advised, as may anti-fungal creams.

Q *Since I returned from travelling round Europe, about a month ago, I've developed this unbearably itchy rash of tiny spots in my armpits, round my belly button and on my bottom and thighs. Have I caught something?*

A This could be scabies, although you should go to your GP for confirmation. Scabies is a tiny mite that burrows under the skin, causing little red spots, often in between the fingers and in the groin area, and also in places such as the elbows, armpits, thighs and stomach. The skin in the affected areas is extremely itchy. The mite is usually transmitted directly from person to person – for example from holding hands, sleeping in the same bed or from sexual contact – but you could have caught it from infested mattresses, even if they looked quite clean. Scabies is treated with permethrin dermal cream (e.g. Lyclear), which is available over the counter, and is very effective and easy to use. You apply it to your whole body, excluding the head and neck, and wash it off 8–12 hours later. Piriton antihistamine tablets (also available over the counter) will ease the itching.

Because scabies is contagious, any people with whom you have been in close contact should be treated too, and you will also need to wash thoroughly all your clothes and bedding. This is sufficient to kill off any stray mites.

Q *I have got an itchy, round, crusty spot on my forearm, about the size of a 10p piece. My wife said I might have caught something from our new puppy, but I think it looks a bit like the eczema I used to have as a child. What can I do about it?*

A Ringworm is a fungal infection that you catch from direct contact with infected animals. Eczema usually causes several patches and is symmetrical, so you would expect to have a similar spot on your other arm. The outer edge of a patch of eczema tends to merge into the surrounding skin, whereas fungal patches like ringworm have a raised edge with a clear area in the middle. You can buy antifungal cream, such as clotrimazole (Canesten) or miconazole (Daktarin), from your pharmacist. If in doubt, ask your GP to take scrapings of the patch and send them to the lab to confirm that it is fungal.

Scaly rash

Q *I have just been told that my dry, scaly rash is psoriasis. I don't know how to cope with it or what to expect. Can you tell me more about it, and is there any way of getting rid of it?*

A Psoriasis is a non-infectious, long-term skin condition in which the cells of the top layer of skin (epidermis) reproduce themselves too quickly, which causes heaped-up cells and inflammation. Psoriasis can be helped a great deal but cannot be cured – although it may eventually burn itself out. It tends to cause dry, scaly patches on the elbows, knees and scalp, which may itch, sting and sometimes bleed. Pitted nails and painful joints may be part of psoriasis.

At least one in every fifty people in the UK has psoriasis at some time in their lives. It can run in families though it is not always inherited. Damaging the skin, or being unwell with an infection such as a sore throat, may trigger psoriasis. Some people find stress, smoking or alcohol can cause the psoriasis to flare up. Studies have shown that the more fruit and vegetables you eat, the less prone you are to psoriasis.

The following remedies have been recommended by some sufferers but no strong evidence can be produced for their effectiveness:

- fish oils
- stress reduction
- stopping smoking
- thermal baths
- acupuncture.

Treatments applied to the skin as creams are usually prescribed by a GP and/or skin specialist. They include:

- moisturisers (e.g. E45) – which help in alleviating the condition but are rarely enough on their own
- coal-tar creams – useful but may sting or stain skin and clothes and have a distinctive smell

- dithranol (Psorin) – similar to coal tar, with the same drawbacks
- steroid creams – good short-term improvement but have side-effects (e.g. skin thinning, wrinkles, easy bruising and loss of colour) and limited usefulness in the long term
- vitamin D derivatives, e.g. calcipotriol (Dovonex) – better than coal tar and dithranol, easier to use, and have fewer side-effects and more long-lasting effects than steroids
- Tazarotene (Zorac) – is a new treatment that is very effective and has relatively few side-effects. However, it must not be used by women contemplating pregnancy as it is dangerous for the developing baby.

Other treatments include phototherapy: this is similar to a sunbed but with the harmful rays filtered out as much as possible. Drugs taken by mouth, e.g. cyclosporin (Neoral) may be advised for severe cases of psoriasis, but may cause side-effects.

It is also worth getting in touch with self-help groups, including the Psoriasis Association.★

Q *For quite a few years I have had an unsightly area just below my left ankle, on the inner side, that my GP has diagnosed as varicose eczema. He has said that nothing can be done about it, but my wife thinks it could ulcerate if knocked. Have you any advice please?*

A Your wife is right to be concerned. However, you can do much to prevent ulceration. Your problem arises because of high pressure in the veins near the surface of the legs. A protein called fibrinogen leaks out of the veins, causing inflammation and stopping oxygen getting to the overlying skin – which becomes itchy, scaly, dry and stained brown by pigment that is deposited in the skin. If the surface of the skin breaks down or is knocked, an ulcer can result, which may prove difficult to heal.

An important factor in trying to prevent ulcers is to keep the skin moisturised. Aqueous cream and E45 should help as long as you are not allergic to lanolin (sheep's wool fat), which they contain. Vaseline and emulsifying cream are other options that do not contain lanolin. If your skin is very flaky, avoid bubble bath and use a moisturiser as a soap substitute. Unfortunately, there is no cure for the brown staining once you develop it, but you can prevent further staining by using support bandages that help to reduce pressure in the veins. The only problem with support bandages or stockings is that if the blood supply to your feet (via the arteries) is poor, the tight stockings may further restrict the blood flow so that your toes become starved of blood. Your GP should check the pulses in your feet before recommending support hosiery and, if in doubt, can get the blood flow to your feet checked using an ultrasound gadget called a Doppler.

Blisters

Q *For the past couple of years I have suffered from itchy hands and feet and then I develop blister-like lumps which are also extremely itchy. The blisters on my hands are usually only visible on close inspection; however the ones on my feet can become quite big. The itch eventually dies away but I am left with areas of dead skin which flake off. I also get cold sores and have an underactive thyroid. What could it be?*

A This condition sounds like pompholyx, which is a type of eczema that affects the soles of the feet and palms of the hands. It is probably unrelated to your cold sores. An underactive thyroid (see Chapter 1) can make your skin generally itchy, but would not account for the blisters that you describe. You can control pompholyx by using plenty of moisturisers, avoidance of anything that seems to exacerbate it (e.g. chemicals in contact with your hands) and steroid ointments when it is bad. Betnovate or Dermovate ointments are the strongest available and are best used three times a day for just a few days at a time. Put the ointment on at night and then a pair of cotton gloves and socks on top to keep the ointment in contact with your skin.

Spots

Possible causes of pustules (pus-filled spots)

Acne

Boils

Herpes (cold sores)   (See Chapter 10)

Impetigo   A bacterial skin infection, often of pre-existing spots or cuts. Results in yellow, crusty spots with a head of pus

Rosacea   A skin condition causing facial flushing, broken blood vessels and tiny spots

---

Possible causes of papules (small raised lumps)

Acne

Warts

Scabies   (See pages 226)

Molluscum contagiosum   (See Chapter 11)

Skin tags

Q *I am 27 years old and have suffered from persistent spots for the last ten years. I've tried many different products, none of which has worked. I keep my skin very clean, eat plenty of fruit and vegetables and avoid caffeine and excessive amounts of alcohol, but my skin is constantly spotty. What else can I do about it?*

A Although it is clearly good for your general health to have a healthy diet, there is no relationship between diet and acne. You could try antibiotic lotions that are applied directly to the skin, e.g. erythromycin (Stiemycin), or oral antibiotics, e.g. minocycline (Minocin), which are available on prescription only. But if your acne is severe or very long-standing, ask for a referral to a dermatologist to get isotretinoin (Roaccutane). This drug gets a bad name because it causes cracked lips and dry, peeling skin that can feel as if you have been sandblasted. You must not get pregnant while on it or for a month after finishing the course. However, it works.

One type of contraceptive pill, Dianette, is good for acne because it counteracts the hormone testosterone, which contributes to greasy skin and spots.

Q *I have suffered from spots and blackheads on my face ever since my teens, and over the years my skin has become scarred. Around my jawline I find my spots are large and become big lumps that don't erupt and are painful. What are these and why am I getting them? They are awful.*

A You may have a form of acne that produces cysts. Trying to squeeze these spots will result in infection and scarring and will not help the problem. Acne can be helped a great deal, and treatments range from benzoyl peroxide (Panoxyl) lotion or cream, which helps blackheads and can be bought over the counter, or very strong medication taken by mouth called isotretinoin (Roaccutane – see above), which can only be prescribed by a skin specialist, and which causes red skin and dry, chapped lips.

In between these two extremes are antibiotics either as creams, lotions or taken orally, which can be prescribed by your GP.

Q *I used to be severely afflicted by acne; it was the bane of my life. The spots have almost gone now, but I still have lots of blackheads across my nose, chin and forehead. I have tried squeezing them, steaming them and the extraction methods. My girlfriend thinks I should try a facial cleanser or even see a beautician. Is there anything I can do to get rid of these blemishes?*

A Blackheads are caused by pores blocked with sweat and oils, not dirt. Picking and squeezing does not help except in the short term. If you do not fancy seeing a doctor, you could follow your girlfriend's advice and see a beautician in a salon. A range of treatments for blackheads will be on offer there, including facials, sauna and extraction using a special blunt instrument that can gently squeeze the blackhead without introducing bugs or damaging the skin.

Q *I have got a pimply sore rash round my bikini line. As a result I can't wear my new high-cut swimsuit when I go on holiday next week. What can I do?*

A The irritation could have been caused by recently shaving or waxing around your groin in preparation for the holiday. If the rash consists of little red pimples, but no yellow, pus-filled spots, try a mild steroid cream, e.g. hydrocortisone (Efcortelan), available on prescription only, although other hydrocortisone preparations are available over the counter. If the rash is yellow pustules, the spots could be infected and you need an antibacterial cream or ointment, e.g. fusidic acid (Fucidin), available on prescription only. If shaving or waxing is the culprit, try a hair-removing cream, such as Immac, instead. This may cause less irritation but you should be careful that it does not get into your vagina as it may cause nasty inflammation.

Using a disposable razor each time you shave reduces the risk of infection, which is what causes the small pus-filled spots.

Thrush (see Chapter 5) in the groin creases can also cause itchy, red rashes and will respond best to an antifungal cream, such as clotrimazole (Canesten). If in doubt, ask your GP.

Freckles, moles, discolouration and skin cancer

Common types or causes of skin discolouration (macules)

Freckles or birthmarks

Chloasma Large patch of pigmented skin, often caused by hormonal changes

Viral illnesses

Allergy/drug reaction

Possible causes of lumps

Sebaceous cyst Fluid-filled swelling in the sebaceous glands (which produce a lubricating fluid) of the skin

Lipoma Fat lump

Xanthoma Cholesterol lump

Skin cancer Basal cell, squamous cell or melanoma (see below)

Q *In my youth, I had a large eagle tattooed on my chest with my then girl-friend's initials. I'm desperate to have it removed now. Is there any reliable way of having it done?*

A Removing a tattoo used to be a real problem. But the advent of lasers has improved treatment no end. Some people still opt to have their tattoo cut out, and plastic surgeons or dermatologists will be able to advise about that. Small tattoos can often be cut out and the skin re-stitched so you are left with only a small scar to show for your mistake. But larger tattoos often occupy too big an area for the cut ends to be simply sewn back together and then it becomes necessary to do a skin graft which may not heal properly, can become infected and may leave a large and cosmetically unacceptable scar.

The use of laser is altogether a better option nowadays but the process may require several treatments and should be done only by a dermatologist or cosmetic surgeon skilled in tattoo removal. A wide range of lasers is used for the different colours. The laser, which is a concentrated beam of light, breaks the ink down into tiny particles which are mopped up by the body's immune system. The laser emits its high energy light in short, sharp bursts which minimises the risk of damaging normal surrounding skin. It does not hurt though you may feel a sharp sting on the skin. The overall effect will depend partly on your skin colour; the darker your colour, the harder it may be to get a good result.

Skin blemishes

Q *I know I'm being vain, but for my fortieth birthday I want to treat myself and get the age spot on my cheek removed. It's a brown mark, like a giant freckle, and I loathe it. How do I go about getting it removed, and is the procedure safe?*

A The thing you must bear in mind is that removing any skin spot may result in a scar that you like even less than the original blemish. The two methods that would be offered to you would be laser or freezing it off with liquid nitrogen. Either technique may result in a darker or paler spot than the rest of your skin. Another option would be to use lots of sunblock on your spot, while letting the rest of your face tan to the same colour as the spot (although of course sun exposure can increase your risk of skin cancer).

Camouflage make-up is also worth considering – or you could just decide that you are probably the only person who notices it, and that it does not really spoil your looks anyway. If you are determined to have it removed, make sure the person wielding the laser or liquid nitrogen is experienced in this type of treatment, and try to get some personal recommendations. This is best done by a doctor trained in these techniques.

(See Chapter 1 for more about cosmetic surgery.)

Q *In the last two months I have developed large brown patches on my face. They have been linked to the contraceptive pill, which I have now stopped taking. Will the patches now go?*

A These patches are chloasmae – increased skin pigmentation that usually develops on the forehead and cheeks. It tends to be hormonally related and some women find it develops when they go on the pill, whereas for others it appears for the first time in pregnancy. Some women notice their faces get a bit darker just before a period. The reason may be an increase in hormones that stimulate the cells that contain the skin's pigment (melanocytes). The patches tend to fade in time but may never disappear entirely. If you are careful to put sunblock on the patch, at least it will not become any darker if and when you go out in the sun. The patch can be disguised with camouflaging make-up such as a tinted moisturiser.

Q *I have flat, brown spots on my face, like big freckles, which have appeared over the years and seem to be getting larger. Is there anything I can do about them?*

A These flat, brown areas of skin are sunspots, and are not cancerous or dangerous, but can be unsightly. They develop on areas exposed to the sun, such as the cheeks, hands and throat, and may gradually enlarge. The best treatment is with a laser, and causes a stinging sensation like a quick slap across the face. After treatment, you feel like you have been sunburned and a scab develops but heals after a couple of weeks, leaving the skin as normal. You will be told to be sure to use sunblock on the treated areas.

Q *I lived in Australia when I was a little girl and have always loved having a tan. When I came to the UK I began using a sunbed. Perhaps as a result my skin is covered with small pale spots rather like scar tissue. I believe these are the result of a loss of melanin, under mosquito-bite and pimple scars. I have tried pure Vitamin E and other creams on my skin, and even thought of fake tanning solutions to even out the colour. Is there something more permanent? I feel so stupid now – all this for the sake of a tan.*

A You can get areas of paleness due to loss of melanin as you say, in any area of skin which has been inflamed or damaged. This is known as post-inflammatory depigmentation. Sometimes it recovers so when you are next in the sun, your skin tans evenly and the pale spots are no longer apparent. You should seriously consider limiting your exposure to the sun and sunbeds; the rays can age the skin and can cause long-term damage, including an increased risk of skin cancer. Make-up is your best bet if you want an even look to your skin. These pale spots are probably far more obvious to you than to anyone else; you could choose to ignore them and highlight other features of your face such as your eyes, using make-up, so the spots are even less noticeable.

Skin cancer

Q *I've got freckles and moles all over me. I'm forever checking them to make sure I haven't got skin cancer, but I'm not sure what I'm checking for. How would I know if any of them were turning malignant?*

A Freckles are small and generally only come out when the sun does, fading away as winter looms (although some people have them all the time). As long as they stay less than 5mm across, you do not need to worry about them at all.

Moles appear in childhood or adolescence and can be flat or slightly raised with a hair sticking out of them.

We all worry about moles becoming cancerous, but melanomas (cancers of the melanocytes), though on the increase, are still rare with 3,500 cases a year in the UK. However, it is worth being vigilant because the more promptly they are treated, the better the outcome.

Some families are genetically predisposed to melanomas and have moles that differ from the rest of the population's. These moles are called dysplastic naevi, and if you have them you should be under the observation of a dermatologist, who can photograph and record all your moles so any changes can be detected. It may be hard to determine whether your moles fall into this category and it is best to see a dermatologist if you are in doubt. Dysplastic naevi are bigger than most moles and more numerous than usual, with 40 or more on the body, are found on parts of the body that ordinary moles do not reach – such as the scalp – and have an irregular outline so they seem to fade into the surrounding skin.

Melanomas are most common on the lower leg of fair-skinned people over 30, but anyone can get one anywhere at any time. They can appear on normal skin and not only as the development of a mole.

If any pigmented (i.e. brown/black) spot on your skin has one of the following characteristics, you should keep an eye on it. If it has two or more of these features you should seek medical advice:

- asymmetrical spot (i.e. not round/oval)
- border irregular
- colour not uniform
- diameter greater than 5mm.

Any pigmented spot that bleeds, itches, or causes you concern should also be checked out. If in doubt, ask your GP – it is best to err on the side of caution.

Q *In recent years I have had ten moles removed. They were suspected of being cancerous. Two did turn out to be cancerous, and in both cases they have been non-life-threatening basal cell carcinomas. All the removals have left me*

Skin cancer

Skin cancer is one of the most common cancers throughout the world. There are three main types: basal and squamous cell cancers and melanomas. Basal cell cancers account for more than half of all incidences of skin cancer; one-quarter are squamous cell cancers, and the remainder include melanomas and other rare types of the disease.

Exposure to the sun is the single biggest risk factor for developing skin cancer, and short bursts of over-exposure to the sun are more dangerous than regular, moderate exposure. People with dark skins are not usually affected by skin cancers, and the vast majority of skin cancers, except melanomas, occur on the head and neck. Most cases occur in people over the age of 30, and women are more susceptible to the disease than are men.

Basal and squamous cell cancers used largely to affect elderly people, although owing to increasing exposure to sunburn, they are becoming more common among younger people. They are usually readily treatable with surgery and/or radiotherapy. Squamous cell cancers are more dangerous than basal cell cancers. Melanomas are less common than basal and squamous cell cancers, but they are potentially more dangerous.

- **Basal cell carcinoma (also known as rodent ulcer)** is rare in people under 50 but increasingly common after that age. Rodent ulcers can grow, but they never spread to other organs and never cause death. They usually crop up on the face, especially near the eyes. Initially *with unpleasant visible scarring. Now the consultant wants to remove two more suspect moles but I am reluctant. What should I do?*

A You have got two different and unrelated skin problems. Basal cell carcinomas (BCCs), also known as rodent ulcers, are usually readily identifiable by doctors and need to be removed by cutting, scraping, freezing or burning. You also seem to have a lot of moles that obviously need watching to ensure that you are not developing a melanoma. Melanomas are not life-threatening if you catch them early (if they are less than 0.85mm deep) but they rapidly become more dangerous as they extend deeper into the skin. That

they look like a small, raised, skin-coloured, glistening lump. Later they look like small ulcers with a rolled edge. They must be treated otherwise they gradually destroy surrounding and underlying tissue. Treatment involves freezing, burning or surgically removing the lump.

- **Squamous cell carcinoma** is also a common cancer which does not usually spread to other organs but can cause nasty damage to surrounding skin. However, if spread does occur, it can be very severe and difficult to treat. These cancers usually occur on the lower lip, rims of the ears and in the mouth. They can look like small nodules or ulcers. They are usually cut out or treated with radiotherapy.

- **Malignant melanoma** attracts more attention than the other types of skin cancer because it is more serious. Every ten years, the incidence of melanoma is doubling. Fair-skinned women exposed to the sun are most at risk, and very rarely, melanoma may run in families who have numerous birthmarks. There are various features that may suggest that a new or existing mole is a melanoma (see above). Treatment involves cutting out the melanoma. No further treatment is required unless the melanoma is advanced. The survival rate is good for people with early melanomas which have not invaded the skin deeply. Once the melanoma spreads to lymph nodes, the survival rate decreases. If it spreads to the liver or other organs, the outlook becomes very poor.

(See Chapter 1 for more about cancer.)

is why the consultant has erred on the side of caution – scars are safer than missing a treatable melanoma. Monitor your own moles: look out for changes of colour and size in them, and for any itching, bleeding or crusting which can be early signs of melanoma.

You could ask to have all your moles photographed regularly so that any changes could be measured.

Q *I have a basal cell carcinoma on the end of my nose. I am trying to find out the very best method of treatment with the least scarring. What do you suggest?*

A Basal cell carcinomas (BCCs) need to be removed because they tend to enlarge and eat away at surrounding tissues. The British Association of Dermatologists recommends seeing a specialist for BCCs on and around the nose, rather than letting your GP remove them, because they tend to recur unless fully destroyed. They can be cut off, scraped ('curettage'), burnt off or destroyed using laser or radiotherapy. All methods, including laser, may leave a scar but it is usually fairly minimal and far less unsightly than an untreated BCC. Remember to use sunblock in future and limit your exposure to the sun – BCCs are more common in fair-skinned people and related to episodes of sunburn and cumulative time spent in the sun.

Veins

Broken veins and capillaries

Q *I am in my late 20s, and within the last six months I've begun to get fine thread veins on my cheeks. They are not too bad at the moment, but the probability that they are going to get worse is making me very worried. Is there anything I can do to stop them getting worse – and possibly remove the ones I already have?*

A Tiny thread veins in the cheeks come on with age. Some of us are more prone to them than others and too much sunbathing makes them worse. Rosacea, a skin condition causing facial flushing and tiny pustules, can result in lots of tiny thread veins as can prolonged steroid treatment. But most people just get a few tiny ones on the cheeks, starting in their late twenties, and gradually increasing with age though rarely to a very noticeable extent. You can get them treated with a laser by a dermatologist or cosmetic surgeon. The surgeon will usually do a test area first. The procedure does not hurt; it feels like a rubber band being flicked against your face. There can be extensive bruising after treatment but it settles quickly. One treatment is usually enough, but if you have a large area to treat, it will probably be spread over a few sessions. The treatment will not be available on the NHS unless the problem is due to rosacea or steroids, because it is deemed to be a cosmetic procedure. The price depends on who does it and the extent of the work, but expect at least £175 for consultation and one-off treatment. (See Chapter 1 for more about cosmetic surgery.)

Q *What can I do about all the broken blood vessels on my thighs, which are really bothering me?*

A These red 'spiders' appear on many women's thighs, noses and cheeks as they get older. Some are more prone to spiders than others, as it may be due to an inherited tendency, sun and wind damage, drinking too much alcohol or previous injury. They do occur in men too, but are less common.

Treatments include:

- **sclerotherapy** – a very fine needle is inserted into the centre of the spider and an irritant solution injected which makes the spider shrivel up. It leaves a little bump which disappears after a few weeks. Further treatment may be needed six weeks later. It is not always successful, and costs around £200
- **electrolysis** – a small electrical current is passed through a needle inserted into the centre of the spider. It may leave a small scar or even cause more spiders to develop. The cost is from £20
- **laser (pulse-dye laser) treatment** – this involves a few sharp pricks, causes some bruising, swelling and numbness but produces by far the best results. It is available from dermatologists only, unlike electrolysis which may be available at beauty clinics. It costs around £250.

Varicose veins

Q *I have very unpleasant and sore varicose veins that ache at the end of each day and look so unsightly that I can't wear shorts or even knee-length skirts in the summer. Should I have them treated and what does the treatment involve?*

A Varicose veins can be unsightly and may ache and throb. When the valves in veins become leaky and do not work properly, blood pools in the veins and the pressure in the veins rises. The veins become elongated, widened and twisty.

You do not have to have them treated unless you want to but they may well get worse as the years go by. Varicose veins can bleed, itch, become inflamed and painful (thrombophlebitis), cause a brown staining of your skin as blood leaks out of them (varicose eczema), and lead to varicose ulcers.

Treatment includes:

- wearing support stockings
- taking regular exercise and raising your legs when you can
- having compression sclerotherapy – an injection of a solution into the vein that blocks off the vein
- having surgery – tying off small veins and stripping out the larger veins in more severe cases. How soon you recover from the operation depends on the extent of the surgery. This surgery is available on the NHS if you need the treatment for more than just cosmetic reasons.

Stretch marks

Q *I am a man in my thirties and recently lost a great deal of weight. I have very unsightly pinkish stretch marks all over my belly. Is there anything I can do about them?*

A Congratulations for having lost so much weight and commiserations about the marks. Stretch marks often appear when you lose or gain weight rapidly. The damage occurs in the deeper layers of your skin, affecting the collagen and elastin which keep skin stretchy. Stretch marks are red or purple at first as deep blood vessels show through the stretched skin, and ideally this is when you should get them treated. Laser can be used to break up the red colour though the skin may not appear normal afterwards but have streaky whitish lines. As the stretch marks fade, they look white or yellowish as the fat in the skin shows through. Some people are more prone to stretch marks than others. The marks can appear at any time, but especially when there are rapid changes to your body shape – for instance, during the pubertal growth spurt and pregnancy. Steroid drugs and medical conditions (e.g. Cushing's syndrome) which cause an increase in normal steroid levels can result in stretch marks.

Keeping your skin well moisturised and avoiding rapid changes to your body shape when possible can help to minimise the risk of stretch marks. Creams and oils which are marketed as being particularly good at treating stretch marks often make rather extravagant claims. Although they may contain collagen, it is doubtful whether the collagen can be absorbed through the skin into the deeper layers and repair the damage that has already been done. Laser treatment once stretch marks have faded to white is often disappointing. Using camouflage make-up or fake tanning may do the trick if you are particularly self-conscious about your stretch marks.

Wrinkles

Q *I hate my wrinkled face, which makes me look much older than I am – I am in my late forties but in my youth I spent too much time sunbathing and using sunbeds. Is there anything I can do about it?*

A You are quite right that sunbathing and using sunbeds may have caused damage to your skin. Exposure to the sun, smoking and genetic factors determine how wrinkled our skin gets, so to avoid wrinkles, it is best to stay out of the sun, use moisturisers regularly and sunblock and protection when in the sun, and not smoke.

In your case, you can avail yourself of the following treatments for your wrinkles.

- **Botulinum toxin injections**, which cause temporary muscle paralysis. The solution is injected into the facial muscles to relax frown lines in the forehead and crow's feet around the eyes. The treatment lasts for about three to six months and then has to be done again. If the treatment is too effective it can result in over-paralysis, causing a startled appearance, and if the injections go into the wrong muscles the eyebrows may droop. These effects too wear off after three to six months. The cost varies, depending on the number of sessions and the extent of the wrinkles.

- **Dermabrasion**, which is a way of smoothing down skin to get rid of fine wrinkles and scars from old acne or chickenpox. Under a local or general anaesthetic, depending on the extent of the work to be done, the skin is 'sanded' down using a small rotating brush instrument. The newly exposed skin is delicate, red and sore. You will need to use an effective moisturiser regularly and keep out of the sun. The skin may become pale, blotchy, scarred and shiny. The cost is around £400.

- **Collagen injections**, which can get rid of furrows, pits, grooves and wrinkles. Collagen is the stuff that binds our bones, skin, muscles and ligaments, and the loss of collagen in our skin over the years is what makes wrinkles appear. Collagen is made up into a paste with salt water and, once injected into wrinkles, the salt water is absorbed, leaving the collagen in place. Two or three treatments may be needed to fill out a wrinkle. Injections may be painful, and local anaesthetic cream can be rubbed on to the area about half an hour before the injection to lessen pain. Allergic reactions causing hard, red, itchy blotches may develop after the injection and take months to disappear. The effects of the injections last for up to six months, then you return to your pre-injection state. The cost is around £300 per session.

- **Laser skin re-surfacing**, which uses a laser to vaporise outer layers of the skin. When the skin heals, surface wrinkles and small scars may be obliterated. It may cause sore skin and scarring.

    (See Chapter 1 for more about cosmetic surgery.)

Hair

Too much hair in the wrong places, too little in the right places, too thick or too thin – hair can be our crowning glory, but is often a source of anxiety and discontent. While men may lament their receding hairlines, many women spend a great deal of time and money fighting a battle against their body hair. Patterns of hair growth vary enormously from one individual to another, and one of the simplest ways of dealing with yours may be to accept it. However, unusually excessive hair growth or loss can cause embarrassment and distress, and if this is the case there are medical options that can help.

Changes in hair growth and hair quality may occasionally signal internal disease, so do not be reluctant to seek medical help if you are concerned about any hair problems.

Hair loss

Possible causes of hair loss
Male pattern baldness
Alopecia
Ringworm   In the scalp, this fungal infection can temporarily weaken or destroy the hair follicles, creating a bald patch
Seborrhoeic dermatitis   (See page 225)

Q *I am a 28-year-old woman, in good general health, but I have been losing my hair for the last four years. It is thinning at the sides and on top and my hairline is receding. I have had a number of blood tests, all normal, except for a check on my hormone levels. My doctor refuses to do this test as my periods are OK. However, I have read that female baldness/hair loss can be caused by a very slight increase in the level of testosterone. Have you any advice on the next steps I could take to alleviate this embarrassing problem?*

A Your hair loss sounds as if it is the type known as male pattern baldness (i.e. receding hairline and a bald patch developing). In men, this is linked to the male hormones, androgens. In women, it is unclear whether hormones do play a part. It is often an inherited tendency, especially in women. The most practical solution is to take the oral contraceptive pill, Dianette, which blocks the male hormones (androgens) and so can help prevent further hair loss. If you cannot take the pill for some reason (e.g. because you have had a thrombosis) or you prefer not to, you could try minoxidil (Regaine) lotion, available over the counter. You have to keep using it or any hair regrowth tends to fall out again, which can prove very expensive.

If you are approaching the menopause then you may want to consider HRT which may halt the process and restore some hair thickness. A blood test will not tell you much but can let you know whether you are approaching the menopause despite regular periods. (See Chapter 6 for more about the contraceptive pill and the menopause.)

If no particular cause is found, advice from a skilled hairdresser is best. There are many commercial sources of help with hair problems but you need to be a little sceptical and careful before spending lots of money on untested or unproven wonder cures.

Q *I know it is normal for men to suffer from thinning hair, but my hair has suddenly started falling out at an alarming rate. I have long hair and when I get out of the bath these days there are great clumps of it left behind. I am only 25. What could be causing it?*

A We shed hair all the time but it looks most obvious and alarming in the bath. Hair thinning may be due to an underlying iron deficiency. A blood test which specifically measures the amount of iron in your body is important, as iron levels can be low enough to cause hair thinning but not low enough to cause anaemia, and a simple full blood count, which is the standard test for anaemia, may miss milder iron deficiency. Iron supplements can restore iron levels to normal and may help you hair to recover its previous thickness.

Hair thinning can also be caused by ill health, anaemia, or a thyroid problem (See Chapter 1).

Dandruff

Q *What works best for dandruff? My wife's always brushing my shoulders and buying me new shampoos from the chemist. It can be very embarrassing sometimes.*

A Two shampoos available over the counter are worth a try: Selsun and Nizoral. They work in different ways so try one first and switch if you have no joy. If your dandruff is accompanied by scaly skin patches, you may have psoriasis (see earlier in this chapter). It is worth a visit to your GP to discuss options in that case.

Excess and unwanted hair

> ### Common causes of excess body hair
>
> **Ethnic origin** Women from Mediterranean and Indian subcontinent countries naturally have more body hair than Nordic women
>
> **Polycystic ovary syndrome (PCOS)** A condition which may cause excess hair, acne, and irregular periods (see Chapter 5)
>
> **Anorexia** Excess hair can result from a relative excess of male hormones (androgens), as the ovaries become inactive (owing to starvation) and the level of oestrogen falls
>
> **Menopause** As above, caused by the falling level of oestrogen
>
> **Drugs** Some drugs, e.g. phenytoin (Epanutin) (anti-epilepsy), danazol (Danol) (hormonal treatment for heavy periods, etc.), and steroids may cause excess hair as a side-effect

Q *I am 36 years old and since I was 22 I started growing facial hair, first on my chin and, after the birth of my children, on my neck and the side of my cheeks. I've tried everything, including bleaching and tweezing, but the results, especially for the chin, are not satisfactory. I am now thinking of laser treatment, but I am not sure whether it is completely safe or effective, especially since it is so expensive. Also, could this problem have its root in a hormone imbalance, and, if so, how could I find out?*

A Your recent growth of facial hair probably does represent a change in your hormonal balance, which is a common phenomenon after childbirth and as you get older. It often occurs after the menopause, when the ovaries produce less and less oestrogen so the male hormones, androgens, which are responsible for hair growth, predominate. Hormonal changes also occur:

- when coming off the contraceptive pill
- after being pregnant
- on some drugs, e.g. steroids (used in severe inflammatory conditions such as asthma).

Losing weight can affect hormonal levels and make hair growth less severe. Dianette, a type of contraceptive pill, is a good option if you need contraception, can take the pill and want to help acne and excess hair.

Laser hair removal requires several treatments, can leave permanent marks and cannot guarantee that the hair will not grow back. Some women have been delighted with the result, others rather disappointed. This treatment is not available on the NHS. Ask your GP to refer you to a consultant dermatologist.

Nails

Most nail problems are a result of previous injury or excessive nail-biting (in which case the nail may grow out discoloured and malformed over the next couple of months), or the nails are misshapen because of a fungal infection. Fungal infections cause thick, crumbly nails, often on one finger or hand only. Oral anti-fungal drugs taken for two to three months will cure most such infections.

Nail problems occasionally signal underlying conditions. For example, skin conditions such as psoriasis cause pitting of the nails of both hands. Some changes in nail shape may be linked to lung or bowel disease. Nails may become spoon-shaped in anaemia, white in diabetes, and yellow in liver disease. So do not hesitate to seek medical advice about any unexplained changes in the appearance of your nails.

Q *I nearly died from pneumonia three months ago and, since my recovery, have noticed lines down all my finger nails. Could I have become deficient in calcium during my illness?*

A The lines in your nails are called Beau's lines and appear several weeks after a very severe illness. They may fade in time or you may be left with them as a legacy of your illness. They do not mean that you are still unwell or signify any vitamin or calcium deficiency. In fact, contrary to popular belief, nail changes do not usually point to deficiencies.

Q *I have small pits in my finger nails. What could be causing them?*

A Pits are small depressed areas of the nail. If they are arranged in a very uniform way, it can be linked with alopecia areata, in which you develop hair loss or a bald patch as part of an auto-immune reaction (when the body reacts against some part of itself, for reasons which are not fully understood). Irregular pits may be linked to psoriasis, which causes scaly patches on the skin and scalp. Pitting may also be part of eczema of the hands, usually caused by contact with cleaning chemicals and other irritants. There is no specific treatment for pitting of the nails but identifying and treating associated conditions may be useful.

(See earlier in this chapter for more about eczema and psoriasis.)

Q *My toenails have become gradually discoloured over the past ten years and are now a brownish colour, which I cover up with brightly coloured nail varnish. What is causing this discolouration?*

A Using nail varnish over long periods of time can make your nails brownish. Dyes from shoes or socks staining your toenails is another common cause of discoloured toenails. Potassium permanganate soaks used to treat infections stain the nails brown.

In the first instance, you should stop using the nail varnish. If you are well and not on any medication, it is unlikely that there is any dangerous cause of your brown nails.

Q *The sides of my nails frequently get painful, red and swollen, and the bottom of my nail near the cuticle has become thick, red and overgrown. I was prescribed oral antibiotics when pus began oozing out of the side of the nail. What could it be?*

A Your condition is known as chronic paronychia and is often related to having your hands in water for long periods of time. The key thing is to keep your hands as dry as possible by avoiding contact with water (try wearing cotton-lined rubber gloves when you do the washing up) and drying your hands carefully after they have been wet. You may be able to avoid further infection by using an antifungal ointment or cream, e.g. clotrimazole (Canesten).

Chapter 10

Head and sense organs

We all get headaches, and many of us suffer from migraine or spells of dizziness. More often than not, these do not indicate anything serious. However, they can be persistent, recurring, and depressing – and because the symptoms relate to our brains, it is quite normal to feel anxious and to fear the worst. Pains in the head, face or neck that result from nerve problems can be equally disturbing, as well as debilitating.

In many cases the cause of such complaints is identifiable, and they can be treated. However, the symptoms can be hard to describe precisely, and the problem is sometimes difficult to diagnose. You may need to discover your own symptom-managing techniques, perhaps involving changes to your lifestyle or the use of complementary therapies that you find suit you.

Our sense organs, in contrast, are less mysterious – and problems such as styes, cold sores, blocked noses or twitching or watery eyes are less likely to provoke fears of fatal illness than to embarrass us by making us look unattractive. However, when senses that we have always taken for granted and on which we depend, such as our sight and hearing, start to let us down, it can be frightening. It might even be such a worry that we feel scared to seek medical advice and ignore the problem in the hope that it will go away.

This chapter discusses possible causes of and treatments for the head problems described above. It looks at sensory concerns such as blurred vision and tinnitus, and gives advice on what you can do about unsightly or embarrassing afflictions such as cold sores, blocked noses or postnasal drip. It also offers practical suggestions about how to deal with snoring.

Glossary

Adenoids   Small patches of infection-fighting (lymphoid) tissue at the back of the nose, which usually shrink by the age of seven

Alexander technique   Teaches self-awareness of body and posture, especially of the head, and also good standing, sitting and walking. Helpful for back problems

Conjunctivitis   Inflammation of the lining of inner part of eyelid and eye (conjunctiva)

Cranial osteopath   An osteopath specialising in bones of the skull and their relationship to health. Manipulation of the skull (cranium) is used to treat a variety of conditions including sinusitis, facial pain and low back pain

ENT   Ear, nose and throat

Gingivitis   Inflammation of the gums, causing bad breath (see also Chapter 8)

Glaucoma   Increased pressure in the eyeball

Ophthalmologist   Eye surgeon

Oral surgeon   An expert in conditions of the jaw and mouth, who has usually trained as a doctor and dentist

Nasal polyps   Fleshy, non-cancerous growths inside the nose associated with allergies; may contribute to snoring

Neuralgia   Pain from a nerve; cause usually unknown

Neurologist   Specialist in diseases of the nervous system

Postnasal drip   Mucus from the nose and sinuses drips down the back of the throat, causing runny nose

Rhinitis   Inflammation of the lining of the nose causing runny nose; caused by allergy or infection

Sinusitis   Inflammation of the lining of the spaces inside the front of the skull

Head

The brain, as well as determining mood and behaviour, is also the nerve centre controlling all vital functions. Headaches usually signal a need to modify your lifestyle in some way: to have a nap, eat, drink, or get up from the computer for a few minutes. Very occasionally, though, they can be a sign of serious underlying disease, and if your headaches seem unusually persistent, severe or are accompanied by other symptoms, such as loss of balance or vomiting, it is always worth seeking medical help.

Headaches

Q *I suffer from headaches practically every day. They are quite incapacitating and last for up to three hours. My GP always takes my blood pressure, says it's OK, and advises paracetamol. I have a lingering fear that I may have a brain tumour, and really feel that I should have a CT scan. Should I insist on one?*

A Headaches are universal; brain tumours rare. But that does not stop all of us worrying, from time to time, that we have one lurking in our heads. And the fact is that brain tumours often go unrecognised in their early stages so, in a sense, we are right to worry. Warning signs of a brain tumour include:

* pain worst in mornings
* early-morning vomiting
* neurological problems, such as loss of vision
* recently-starting headaches, once over the age of 50, having never been a headache sufferer before.

Most headaches are due to migraine (see below) or trapped nerves in the neck. High blood pressure does not cause headaches, unless it is exceptionally high. But if you have any of the warning signs, you could ask your GP to refer you for a CT or MRI (magnetic resonance imaging) scan to set your mind at rest. However, a CT or MRI scan will only be requested by a neurologist if there is a significant risk of your having a brain tumour or a serious underlying problem.

Q *When I am active I have sharp pains, like electric shocks, across the top of my head – as if my brain has difficulty processing enough oxygen. What is causing this problem and is it something to worry about? Should I give up physical activity, or should I try to exercise through the pain in order to keep fit?*

A Your sharp pains sound very much like tension headaches, although if you have any of the warning signs of a brain tumour (see above) it would be a good idea to be checked over by a neurologist to be certain. We all get headaches from time to time and the things that we worry about when we get a severe, unexplained or prolonged headache – such as brain tumours, meningitis, or bleeds in the brain – are actually very rare. The most common causes are tension headache, sinusitis, migraine and wear and tear in the neck (cervical spondylosis). It is worth getting your eyes checked to see whether you need glasses, although eye strain is not usually a cause of headaches. Contrary to popular belief, high blood pressure does not cause headaches except in very rare cases when it is phenomenally high.

Tension headaches may be made worse by painkillers, and the first advice would be to stop all painkillers, especially those containing codeine. If you have to take anything, paracetamol in the minimum possible dose is probably best. The advice for tension headaches is basic, common-sense stuff about lifestyle: eat small, regular meals to avoid getting too hungry, drink plenty of fluids, avoid alcohol, and get some fresh air and exercise every day. Some people are helped by acupuncture or cranial osteopathy for this kind of problem.

Q *For several months now I have been experiencing sharp, fierce and frequent headaches. They come quickly when I am doing exercise, such as bike riding, running etc. – as well as when I (attempt to) have sexual intercourse. They go fairly quickly (within 10 mins) once I stop the activity, leaving a slight dull headache behind. It is becoming very depressing and frustrating. What can be done to help?*

A The type of headache you describe is harmless and is a reaction to the activity you are doing. Blood flow is being diverted to your muscles or genitals and chemicals are being released that contribute to the headache. If you do not get headaches at other times and have no visual disturbance or vomiting, you are highly unlikely to have any serious underlying condition. To prevent the headache you may want to approach all these activities more gradually; more gentle foreplay during sex and a slower start to the cycling may help.

Migraine

Q *I am a 32-year-old woman and am suffering for at least two days a month with pain in the face and around, under and above the right eye. I have had other symptoms that have come and gone this year, such as tingling in the fingers and slight slurring of speech – which is quite frightening – lasting for a few minutes. My GP gave me Imigran, saying that it is very good for migraine, and it definitely helped. I am still not convinced that I have migraine and wonder whether there are other causes, and also what I can do about the headaches?*

A Yes, the pain over one eye and temporary speech problem, which then improve with no lasting ill-effects, are most likely to be migraine. Migraine is a condition that is caused by spasm – a short-lived closing, then opening, of blood vessels in the brain. Changes in chemicals in the brain (including one called 5HT) occur at the same time.

Many migraine sufferers find that their migraines are triggered by foods such as wine, cheese or chocolate. Attacks may be worse on the contraceptive pill or before a period. Anxiety, exercise, travel, tiredness and hunger are also sometimes triggers, but 50 per cent of sufferers cannot identify specific triggers.

Migraine can be heralded by an 'aura', lasting around 15 minutes, which causes visual disturbances such as dots or zig-zag lines in front of the eyes, speech difficulties or stumbling around. Within one hour, the throbbing headache starts, which is typically but not always felt over one eye. Nausea, vomiting, unwillingness to look at bright lights, and an inability to do anything may all accompany the headache. Afterwards, you might feel exhausted.

Treatment of migraine includes prevention of attacks by identifying and avoiding potential triggers. If you have slurred speech or loss of sensation down one side, you must avoid the contraceptive pill as there may be an increased risk of strokes (see Chapter 6 for more about this). If you have more than two attacks a month, you may want to take medication to prevent attacks, e.g. amitriptyline (Triptafen) or propranolol (Inderal).

If you do get an attack, you need to lie down in a dark, quiet room if possible. Aspirin or paracetamol, along with a drug to stop nausea and increase absorption of the painkillers, e.g. metoclopramide (Maxolon) or domperidone (Motilium), is the best approach. Drugs like sumatriptan (Imigran) have largely superseded older drugs such as ergotamine (Migril), although Imigran may still not be more effective than painkillers with metoclopramide.

If you are not convinced that you have migraine, and are still worried that you have some nasty underlying problem – a brain tumour, multiple sclerosis or mini-strokes are the three conditions that most people with severe headaches worry about most – share your concerns with your GP, who may well be able to reassure you, or ask for referral to a neurologist to set your mind at rest.

Further information is available from the Migraine Action Association.★ See also Chapter 6.

Dizziness

Q *For some time I have been having spasms of feeling dizzy, as well as feeling exhausted and sick as soon as I get up in the morning and for most of the day. What could be wrong with me?*

A There are several possibilities:

- you may have low blood pressure – when you leap out of bed in the morning, stand for long periods of time or get very hot and bothered it can make you feel dizzy. Low blood pressure is good for you in the long-term, in that you are less likely to get heart attacks or strokes. But it can make you feel rather ill and washed out, so it is worth having your blood pressure measured when you are sitting and when you stand up, to see whether it falls to low levels (e.g. below 90/60). It helps to get up slowly, sit down if you are feeling woozy, drink plenty of fluids, avoid getting too hot and avoid drugs that lower blood pressure, such as diuretics (water pills)
- you could be anaemic (see Chapter 1). Anaemia makes you tired, breathless, pale and exhausted. A simple blood test will tell you whether this is the problem. If you have heavy periods or are breastfeeding, you may be a bit low in iron, which makes you anaemic. Iron tablets for six weeks or more will restore the blood cells and energy
- you may not be eating enough. Low blood sugar levels are rare but if you find that eating restores your energy and that you feel worst just before lunch, that may be a cause

- your thyroid might be underactive. That makes you feel tired, cold a lot of the time, gives you puffy ankles after standing and puffy eyes after lying down, and also prone to put on weight. Again, a blood test can diagnose this too, and thyroid tablets taken daily should improve matters. (See Chapter 1 for more about thyroid problems.)

Q *In the last six weeks I have experienced regular attacks of giddiness and nausea – although the sensation occurs in my head, not my stomach. It feels as if the world is spinning, although visually things remain stationary. The attacks are brought on by my moving my head, and last for a few seconds. My hearing is fine. Movement and even looking around during these attacks makes it worse, and I am left sitting or lying in one fixed position for several minutes, too frightened to move. Is it something serious?*

A The most likely cause of your problem is called benign positional vertigo (BPV). It causes brief but severe attacks of vertigo (dizziness), which come on when you turn your head. It can be caused by a head injury but more commonly comes on after viral illness or as the result of long-term middle-ear infections. Most sufferers learn to avoid turning their head during attacks but obviously that is not always possible. There are formal exercises you can be taught which help relieve the symptoms. Most people get better even without treatment after six months or so. If you also experience hearing loss and ringing in the ears, you may have Menière's disease – a problem in the inner ear which can cause permanent hearing loss. You should ask your GP for a referral to an ENT surgeon for a proper diagnosis and help with the exercises if BPV is the problem.

Pain in the head, face or neck

Q *I have been suffering with a stiff neck, headaches, tingling in my arms and a sensitive scalp for some months. I have had treatment from a physiotherapist but he has now discharged me, saying I need to see a specialist. I work as a lifeguard so I need to stay mobile, and this is having a serious effect on my work and wellbeing. What could be causing the pain?*

A The symptoms you describe are typical of pressure on the nerves that come off the spinal cord in the neck and spread across the scalp and shoulders, and down the arms into the fingers. It may be the way you sit, the way you swim or just the way you are made that is predisposing you to this problem.

An osteopath who is experienced in a technique called cranial osteopathy can be of enormous benefit in freeing up the pressure. If that does not work, painkillers such as paracetamol or ibuprofen (Brufen) will ease the pain. Yoga can increase your suppleness and prevent the problem recurring, and a teacher of the Alexander technique, if you can find one in your area, can look at the way you swim and may be able to suggest changes to your technique to prevent recurrences.

Q *I have severe pain starting just above my left ear and spreading across the left side of my face, which feels like it is burning. I also have pins and needles in the left side of my nose, mouth and around the eye. What could it be?*

A Your condition is called trigeminal neuralgia, which refers to pain in the nerve that comes out of the brain and serves one side of the face. The nerve is split into three parts – the top part supplies the face above the cheekbone, the second part serves the part of the face between the cheekbone and corner of the mouth, and the third part serves the area below that. The neuralgia usually affects one of these three parts. No one knows what causes the condition – it may be a viral infection. The area of the face that is affected becomes acutely sensitive, especially to touch and cold winds. Wrapping up in a muffler or scarf before venturing outdoors is a good idea. The drug carbamazepine (Tegretol) is often prescribed and helps to dull the pain and reduce inflammation in the nerve. The condition tends to improve over a few weeks but does sometimes recur.

Q *I frequently get a pain on the left side of my head, between the ear and the forehead. This last a few seconds, then it goes away and at the same time my neck seems to lock. Do you have any idea what this could be? My doctor just wanted to prescribe antidepressants, which I am not keen on taking.*

A It is quite understandable that you would not want to take antidepressants unless you are depressed. There are a number of possible causes of your pain:

- **jaw pain** – if moving your jaw from side to side brings on the pain, you may be grinding your teeth at night or have a malalignment of your back teeth, which means that you bite awkwardly and put strain on your jaw joint. Your dentist can advise you as to whether this is likely by looking at your back teeth
- **migraine** (see page 252) – usually preceded by a wave of nausea and a sharp pain over one eye, and often leaves you feeling worn out
- **trigeminal neuralgia** (see previous question) – a shooting pain that can be triggered by going out in a cold wind
- **temporal arteritis** – a throbbing pain in the temple, which gets gradually worse and requires urgent medical attention. This is rare in people under the age of 60, and unlikely in your case
- **cervicalgia** – pain in the neck that leads to muscle spasm, which traps the little nerves that leave the spinal cord and supply different areas of the face, scalp or shoulders. You may be sleeping or turning awkwardly and putting pressure on the nerve that supplies your temple. Wearing a neck collar for a couple of days is advised by some doctors and physiotherapists, but prolonged use of a collar may increase stiffness. Some gentle physiotherapy or seeing an osteopath (who uses massage and manipulation to correct posture and aid blood circulation) or chiropractor (who also uses manipulation, but focusing more on the nervous system) should help.

Eyes, ears, nose and mouth

Our sense organs may cause us annoying or cosmetic problems, but in general they serve us very well. Blocked or runny noses, ringing in the ears and mouth ulcers can make our life a misery – but our nose enables us to breathe and smell and is also a major line of defence against intruding bugs; our mouth and tongue are crucial for eating as well as critical for communication; and in addition to enabling us to hear, our ears help to keep us balanced as we move around.

Those of us who are fully-sighted probably rely on our vision more than any other sense. Fortunately, modern medical techniques have made a huge difference to those with eye problems. Eye disease can develop silently, manifesting itself only once extensive damage has been done. Therefore it is important that babies and children with squints, adults with diseases that may affect their eyes (such as diabetes and high blood pressure) and anyone with a family history of glaucoma, have detailed eye examinations.

Eyes

Stye

Q *I have got a stye on my eyelid, which is painful and looks horrible. What can I do about it?*

A These unpleasant little abscesses form at the base of an eyelash. The stye will come to a head, pointing outwards, and will then burst and release its pus within a week. Antibiotic eye ointment such as chloramphenicol (Chloromycetin), available on prescription only, may speed up the process. Brolene and other eye drops available over the counter will not help. If you speak to your GP on the phone, he or she may be happy to leave you out a prescription for collection so you do not have to wait for an appointment. However, treatment is often not necessary as the stye is likely to heal on its own.

Eyelid swelling

Q *I have had a small white swelling on my eyelid for some months. It is not painful but it is unsightly. What is it and can it be treated?*

A It sounds like a meibomian cyst. These start off as a blockage in the meibomian glands, which are tiny glands in the eyelids. The blockage causes a swelling which points in towards the eyeball, rather than outwards like a stye, and does not irritate as much as a stye does. The problem is that unlike a stye, which usually disappears without trace, the meibomian cyst heals leaving a tiny, hard swelling like yours. If it does not bother you, you can leave it alone; but if it does you could ask your GP to refer you to an ophthalmologist to have it cut out. If it swells again and becomes painful, you can put a warm compress of a towel soaked in warm water on it, and apply chloramphenicol (Chloromycetin) eye ointment, which you can get on prescription from your GP.

Growth below the eye

Q *I have what looks like a wart just below my eye. My doctor prescribed some antibiotic cream, which I have been applying for a fortnight, but with no improvement. The wart remains tender and it irritates when I apply the cream. Is this something I should worry about, and is there any alternative treatment?*

A The growth could be a skin tag. These are not infectious or dangerous, but may be unsightly or irritating. If it bothers you, you may want to have it removed. It can be tied at the base with a piece of thread, then burnt, frozen or cut off.

Sagging eyelids

Q *I am seriously considering plastic surgery to have my sagging eyelids done. I am only 30 and feel very self-conscious about them. Could you tell me more about the procedure?*

A Having the excess skin and fat cut away from above and below the eyelids is known as blepharoplasty. The operation is usually done as a day case under general anaesthetic. Discuss it with your GP first to ensure there are no other health problems that may impact on the operation – such as diabetes, high blood pressure or other medical reasons which would make a general anaesthetic dangerous for you, and get your eyes checked by an optician, although the operation should not affect your vision in any way.

However, you will not be able to get this operation done on the NHS if it is for cosmetic reasons, and a decision to opt for cosmetic surgery is not to be made lightly.

(See Chapter 1 for a full account of the pros and cons of cosmetic surgery, and the factors that you should consider before deciding to go ahead with any such operation.)

Twitching eyes

Q *In the last week my right eye has started twitching – lasting for about 30 seconds and recurring every 20 minutes or so. I have worn glasses for over 30 years and have my eyes checked regularly. However, I have been working with a computer for over 15 years. Could this have had an adverse effect on my eyes?*

A Eye twitching worries people but is usually just a sign of tiredness and nothing more. However, it does make sense to have your eyes checked to see whether you need a change to your glasses, and at the same time you could ask the optician to check the pressure in your eyes for the possibility of glaucoma.

At work, make sure that your computer screen does not flicker too much. It is equally important that you sit at the correct distance from your screen, that the screen is at the right height and is tilted and swivelled to a comfortable viewing position. If necessary, fit it with a glare filter. Placing the computer screen out of direct sunlight will help too.

Watery eyes

Q *I am having problems with sore and watery eyes. They run most of the time, which means my make-up looks a mess. I have tried eye drops but these don't seem to be helping. It makes me very self-conscious and is getting me down. What can I do?*

A Irritation of the eyelids and lining of the eyelids (conjunctivae) is very common and is usually caused by make-up, make-up remover or contact lens solutions. The best way to find out what is causing the irritation would be to stop using make-up (including cleansers and moisturisers) altogether and wash your face only with cold water. If you wear contact lenses, take them out and wear glasses for a week instead.

A dab of Vaseline rubbed gently on the eyelids at night and in the morning will help any dry, irritated skin. Do not put any drops in your eyes – you may be allergic to the drops. If you follow this routine and the irritation and weeping stop, you could try using eye make-up (preferably hypoallergenic) gradually, if necessary, with a simple moisturising cream (i.e. an unperfumed, hypoallergenic one) to remove the make-up.

If this routine does not work and your eyes become bloodshot or the skin of your eyelashes is inflamed, you need to see your GP.

Blurred vision

Q *Recently I have been suffering from occasional blurred vision – my eyes can be perfectly clear, then one eye will be blurry for a while. Then it will clear, then one or both will blur over again. It is very worrying. What could it be?*

A Intermittent visual disturbances are always alarming and need to be checked out. However, if your vision clears completely between these episodes of blurred vision, and you are otherwise well, it is likely that you do not have any serious underlying problem and you may never find out exactly what causes the blurring. Possible causes of blurred vision include the following.

- You need **glasses**. The most common cause of blurred vision is that you need glasses or that the ones you have are no longer the right strength. There is a tendency to get more long-sighted as we get older, and many people need glasses for the first time once they get over 40.
- **Cataract**. The most common cause of gradual blurring of vision that is not corrected by glasses. Cataract is due to damage to the lens of the eye, which happens as we age. A short operation, done under local anaesthetic, can literally restore the sight of cataract sufferers.
- **Glaucoma** (see below). Anyone with blurring of vision that is gradually getting worse should be checked for glaucoma by having the pressure inside their eyes measured by an optician or eye specialist.
- **Senile macular degeneration**. A gradual loss of vision in the middle of the visual field, so that you can see things at the side but not straight ahead. More common in very short-sighted people. Laser treatment of the eye can help vision to a certain extent although the continuing deterioration in vision cannot yet be treated successfully.
- Other causes are rare and include alcohol poisoning, diseases of the nervous system, such as multiple sclerosis, and rare inherited conditions that cause visual loss.

For your own reassurance you should have a full medical check-up, including blood pressure measurements and a urine or blood check for diabetes (see Chapter 1), which can cause blurring of vision along with excessive thirst, passing lots of urine and weight loss.

You should also have a detailed eye examination by a reliable optician or referral by your GP to an ophthalmologist. This examination should include checking the pressure in your eyeballs for glaucoma. Glaucoma causes eye pain, blurred vision, haloes around lights (i.e. a blurred area around bright lights) and eventually tunnel vision, which means an inability to see objects at the sides of your visual field.

Q *I recently read an article which linked failing eyesight with kidney disease. I am a relatively heavy drinker and am starting to have slightly blurry vision – could that be the cause? I wear glasses to drive and at the cinema. Could my eyesight be deteriorating naturally or is there a test I could have to establish whether it is my kidneys?*

A Blurred vision is not usually the result of kidney problems, although it can be an early-warning sign of eye problems (e.g. cataract) or a more generalised disease such as diabetes.

The two most common causes of kidney disease are high blood pressure and diabetes. Drinking too much alcohol may make you prone to both, as well as other problems such as stomach ulceration, liver disease and neurological conditions such as tremor, fits and dementia. (See Chapter 1 for more about excessive drinking.)

It is worth paying a visit to your GP for a thorough check-up. He or she can check your blood pressure and do blood tests (urea and electrolytes) that will tell you whether your kidneys are functioning well, whether your liver and blood cells are showing signs of excess alcohol intake, and whether you are diabetic. If there is any concern about your eyes, you can be referred to an ophthalmologist.

It could be that you just need new spectacles, so make an appointment to see an optician. Get the pressure in your eyeballs checked at the same time to rule out glaucoma.

Ears

Tinnitus

Q *I have suffered from intermittent ringing in the ears (tinnitus) for many years, and it is seriously affecting the quality of my life and making me quite depressed. I have spent thousands of pounds (and hours) in search of a cure. Could you tell me whether there is any solid evidence for specific treatments, before I waste any more money?*

A The sad fact is that there is very little good evidence of effective treatments for the debilitating problem of tinnitus. The drug betahistine (Serc) can be helpful in treating dizziness and nausea, although a common side-effect of this drug is that it gives you a dry mouth. There is some evidence, though not much, to support anti-depressants such as amitriptyline (Lentizol) and a Valium-type drug called alprazolam (Xanax) for tinnitus, but both may cause unwanted side-effects. A technique which uses electrical stimulation over the ear may be worth a try, and alternative therapies that are suggested include acupuncture, biofeedback, hypnosis and ginkgo; however, the evidence for their effectiveness is shaky or non-existent.

One cause of tinnitus is Menière's disease, other symptoms of which are dizziness, lack of balance, and hearing loss that may get worse with successive attacks.

There is much work to be done in this underfunded field. The lack of evidence represents a lack of good trials – it does not necessarily mean you should give up trying to find a treatment that could work for you.

You may want to be referred to an expert in audiological medicine (the study of hearing and balance) or an ENT specialist to ensure there is no underlying problem – although it is rare to find any remediable cause of tinnitus. Useful information is available from the Royal National Institute for Deaf People (RNID)★, which has a tinnitus helpline, and the British Tinnitus Association.★

Hearing loss

Q *My elderly father is becoming increasingly isolated. I suspect that he can't hear us and that this is making him reclusive and anti-social. He has got a hearing aid but hates wearing it as he says it is uncomfortable and buzzes. I am worried about his situation. What can I do to help?*

A You can encourage him to ask his GP to refer him back to the hearing aid clinic. NHS hearing aids have in the past been inferior to privately available digital hearing aids, but things are improving now, with an NHS digital hearing aid programme.

The Royal National Institute for Deaf People (RNID)★ has a leaflet called *Equipment for Deaf People*, which lists devices such as special telephones, smoke alarms and doorbells. Your father's GP can also refer him to a hearing therapist to advise about equipment and provide support, a speech and language therapist to help with communication, and a social worker to help tap in to other resources and local support groups. Private hearing aids are supplied by private dispensers, which are monitored by the Hearing Aid Council,★ to whom you can complain if your father gets unsatisfactory service. Another useful organisation is Hearing Concern.★

Nose

Blocked nose

Q *My husband has had a blocked nose for almost two years. He finds it very frustrating and rather embarrassing. Our doctor suggested that he use one of those nasal sprays normally used for colds or 'flu, but it didn't work, and anyway, he never suffers from colds or 'flu. He has a stressful job and I wonder whether this is connected. Do you have any advice?*

A The most common cause of a permanently blocked-up nose is nasal polyps – fleshy swellings inside the nose. These often develop when the lining inside the nose is irritated by an allergy. This might be something that your husband inhales through his nose, such as cat's fur, house-dust mites or pollen in the hayfever season. Allergic reactions cause streaming eyes, sneezing and a runny nose as well as the blocked-up sensation.

Nasal sprays or drops that contain steroids can reduce inflammation of the lining of the nose and even shrink small polyps, but this clearly did not work in your husband's case. The next step would be referral to an ENT surgeon for a closer look up your husband's nose. If he has got large polyps, they can be surgically removed.

The problem is unlikely to be due to stress, although stress may make him focus more on, and worry about, the troublesome symptoms.

Snoring

Q *My partner snores loudly and has done for years. This seems to be getting worse and now wakes me up frequently during the night. Is there a cure? Please help.*

A Snoring is often treated as a bit of a joke. But those of us who sleep with a snorer know that it is no laughing matter.

Snoring is the noise made by vibrations in the roof of your mouth. It occurs most commonly in those people who breathe through their mouth while they are asleep, although it is also possible to snore through your nose with your mouth tightly shut.

Any condition that blocks the flow of air through the nose may produce snoring; for example, a cold or sinus infection, a runny nose caused by allergy to dust, pollen or a particular food, polyps in one or both nostrils, a broken nose or enlarged adenoids. Your nose may also become blocked if the internal lining swells (rhinitis), which can occur as part of an allergic reaction or when you have a viral infection such as a cold. Being overtired, smoking, eating a large meal and drinking alcohol may all make you snore more.

Sleeping on your back increases the chance of snoring because this position encourages your tongue to slip to the back of your throat, partly blocking the air passages.

Simple home remedies for snoring include:

- losing excess weight
- sleeping in a more upright position, on pillows or by raising the head of the bed
- tying a scarf round the head and jaw to stop the mouth dropping open
- stitching a rolled-up sock, tennis ball or cotton reel to the back of your pyjama jacket or nightgown to make it too uncomfortable to sleep flat on your back
- putting a vaporiser in the bedroom, as a dry atmosphere encourages snoring
- cutting down on alcohol and not smoking
- avoiding late evening meals.

See your GP if these measures do not make any difference, or if you notice that your partner regularly appears to stop breathing during the night as well – a condition known as sleep apnoea. The doctor may recommend a plastic device, now available in most large pharmacies, which, by widening the upper part of the nostrils, can improve the air flow and stop snoring. A neck collar can help some snorers by keeping their lower jaw held forward while they sleep.

A surgical operation may be necessary if the underlying cause is a nasal polyp, enlarged adenoids, or if the septum (the wall inside the nose that divides it in two) needs to be straightened. Steroid or decongestant nasal preparations may cure the problem if the nose becomes congested at night, but should not be used for prolonged periods.

Referral to an ENT surgeon for consideration of laser surgery or surgery to the palate is an option, although be warned that, though often successful, there is a certain level of discomfort after the operation and snoring does sometimes restart after a few months.

If snoring is causing daytime sleepiness (either because the snorer is waking him- or herself up, or because he or she is not breathing normally and is retaining too much carbon dioxide, which can cause drowsiness) a CPAP machine can help. The snorer wears a mask over his or her nose during sleep, while a machine pumps in a steady stream of air. The machines often have to be purchased, as few are available on the NHS. They cost £500–600 and should only be considered on the recommendation of an ENT specialist or sleep clinic.

If all else fails, the snorer's partner should buy heavy-duty earplugs.

Postnasal drip

Q *I have suffered from postnasal drip for several years. I've been told that it could be the result of a virus I developed after a bad case of 'flu, and someone else told me that it could be caused by an allergy. This condition is making me quite depressed. What can I do about it?*

A Postnasal drip is the term given to fluid dripping down the back of your nose into the back of your throat. It is due to swelling and excess mucus production in the lining of the nose (rhinitis). This is usually caused by allergies such as hayfever, although it may be hard to identify the allergy. Viruses such as those causing the common cold often make the postnasal drip worse.

As you have had the postnasal drip for a long time, you may want to arrange for an allergy test so that you can avoid the cause if it can be identified – common causes are house dust, cat fur or pollen. Steroid nasal sprays or drops (e.g. Beconase) for ten days at a time or during flare-ups are very effective. Steam inhalations help some people, and antibiotics may be needed from time to time if the nasal discharge becomes thick and green. Some homeopathic treatments may also be effective.

Mouth

Mouth ulcers

Q *For the past two years I have been suffering from chronic mouth ulcers, which seem to appear in cycles every week or so. They occur in different parts of my mouth, often (and most painfully) on my tongue, with as many as five at any one time. I feel worn down and disheartened by the almost constant irritation. Is there anything that will clear them up for good?*

A Although just under a quarter of the population suffer from mouth ulcers, we still do not know much about what causes them. Though troublesome they are almost always harmless, and rarely indicate any specific disease. They can very occasionally be a sign of an underlying disease – most commonly Crohn's disease (see Chapter 7), which causes bowel inflammation, but the other symptoms would be diarrhoea and weight loss.

If you have bleeding gums when you brush your teeth and bad breath (ask your best friend), your ulcers could be linked to gum disease – gingivitis, or, more severely, acute necrotising ulcerative gingivitis (ANUG), also known as trench mouth or Vincent's angina. A swab of the ulcers would show typical cells known as Vincent's organisms. (See Chapter 8 for more about this.)

People with mouth ulcers often think they are vitamin deficient or undernourished in some way, but that is rarely the case. If you have a permanently sore tongue and cracks at the sides of your mouth (see below), in addition to your ulcers, you may be iron deficient, and a simple blood test would pick this up. Other vitamin deficiencies are rare unless you are an alcoholic or have a particularly unusual diet.

If the ulcers are painful white spots, you may have thrush (candida) in your mouth, which can occur if you use steroid sprays for asthma, are on oral steroids, or have impaired immunity due to being diabetic, or have other underlying immune problems. Thrush improves with antifungal lozenges or pastilles (e.g. Nystan).

Unfortunately, however, what you have probably got is known as recurrent aphthous ulceration – which may have a fancy name but has no known cure or cause. In this case it is sensible to avoid trauma to the lining of the mouth, so check for chipped teeth and avoid over-hard brushing. Steer clear of spicy foods, acid fruits such as lemons, and hot drinks while you have the ulcers. Try rinsing your mouth four times a day with a salt mouthwash, using half a teaspoon of salt in a cup of warm water. Triamcinolone (Adcortyl in Orabase) is a paste available on prescription that contains a mild steroid and soothes the soreness.

Cracks at side of mouth

Q *I am 74 years old and am plagued by splits at the sides of my mouth, which become so sore that I have to take my dentures out. It is stopping me from enjoying my food and bothering me a great deal. What could it be, and is there any treatment?*

A This problem, known as angular cheilitis, is most likely to be caused by your dentures. If you do not wear both top and bottom sets regularly or the dentures do not fit well, your upper lip may be over-riding your lower lip, causing deep grooves at the angles of the mouth. Saliva and sweat can collect in the grooves causing infection, usually with thrush (see above). If this is the case, get your dentures checked, always wear both sets and scrub them daily with ordinary soap and water to clear them of candida spores. Vaseline and clotrimazole (Canesten) cream help, and you should use a sun-blocking lipsalve in the sun.

In people who do not wear dentures, this problem may be caused by a number of other conditions. For example, it can be a sign of iron-deficiency anaemia. If you have not had a recent blood test, ask your GP to do one. The blood test will also indicate whether you are deficient in B vitamins or folic acid.

The little cuts can also be associated with Crohn's disease (see Chapter 7), which causes inflammation throughout the gut from mouth to anus. However, if you do not also have diarrhoea and abdominal pains, Crohn's is unlikely. Food allergies would be more likely to make your lips tingle and swell than produce small cuts, so an allergy is unlikely as a cause unless you can clearly link your symptoms to a particular food.

Cold sores

Q *I have an ugly sore at the side of my mouth. It started off with some tingling, and a day later a small cluster of painful blisters developed, which are now, after three days, just beginning to crust over. I have also felt quite run down, as if I had a mild dose of 'flu. I haven't had cold sores before but I think that is what this could be. Please could you tell me more, and what I can do about it?*

A It does indeed sound like cold sores – but you can rest assured that if you do ever get it again, you are unlikely to feel as bad as you did with this first attack.

Cold sores are caused by the herpes simplex virus – a persistent devil of a virus, which tends to recur. Herpes simplex can cause sores anywhere. They are called 'cold sores' on the face, 'whitlows' on the fingers and 'herpes' on the genitals, feet, knees, etc. Most people do not even realise that they have contracted herpes simplex. Blood tests show that most adults have caught the virus at some time in their lives but they have never had symptoms.

Many people are lucky, and after their primary illness they never have further symptoms. A minority have further outbreaks, though these can be often so slight that they do not interfere with daily life. A small number of people have repeated outbreaks, which can range from very painful to just a nuisance. Episodes are often triggered by a lowered immune response, which can be brought about by stress, illness or tiredness. Sunlight on the affected skin is another trigger – especially for facial cold sores. Too much alcohol, cigarettes, and a poor diet are also causes.

You catch the herpes simplex virus by kissing someone who already has the virus, by close facial contact, or by oral sex with someone who has, or has had, genital herpes (even if he or she does not have sores at the time). Thereafter, the virus remains dormant in your system and can resurface any time, especially if you are run down. The minute you feel that tell-tale tingling round your lips that heralds an attack, you can start using acyclovir (Zovirax) cream, or similar anti-viral drugs, which help the cold sores.

(See Chapter 3 for more about genital herpes.)

Chapter 11

Pregnancy and children's problems

Worrying about your children is part of being a parent. It is also something that starts soon after conception – especially if the baby is your first. Of course, many of the fears you might have will be unfounded or irrational, so you may feel reluctant to take them to your doctor. However, anxiety is not good for you or your child: it is important to find out the facts, debunk any myths, and put your mind at rest. It is equally necessary to be aware of anything that could pose a real threat to your offspring.

During pregnancy it is natural to be concerned about any dangers to your unborn baby. Health worries may include the implications of illness in the mother, potential sources of dangerous disease, or genetic abnormalities such as Down's syndrome. Some difficulties that women experience during pregnancy can cause great distress and yet have no obvious medical solution – the most common being morning sickness. You may need help and support if such a problem is making you very unwell.

Once your baby is born – again, particularly if it is your first – you are bound to experience anxieties or fears. A major one is cot death, and you need to know what to do to minimise the risk of this. And almost every parent wonders or worries, at some time or other, whether their child is normal and is developing properly. The safety of childhood vaccinations is another concern – one that has received its fair share of media attention.

School-age children are exposed to a plethora of germs and contagious diseases, some of which you may find quite embarrassing – the classic example being head lice – but no family is immune to such problems, and no child survives his or her school years without the odd childhood illness. The social obstacles of those years in the playground may be more of a worry, however. If you suspect that your child is being bullied, or have received complaints about his or her behaviour towards other children, it can be extremely upsetting and hard to know what to do or where to get help in dealing with the situation.

Although it is impossible to cover the huge range of health worries relating to children in such a short space, this chapter addresses the common ones, including all those mentioned above. The advice offered should aid your understanding and guide you in seeking further help and professional support where necessary. Details of useful organisations are given at the back of the book.

(See Chapter 2 for more about disorders such as autism, Asperger's syndrome and obsessive-compulsive disorder. For more general information, see *The Which? Guide to Children's Health*.)

Childline★ is a helpline available to children or young people in danger or distress.

Pregnancy

Tips for a healthy pregnancy

- Take folic acid from when you stop using contraceptives until the twelfth week of your pregnancy, to reduce the risk of spina bifida and related conditions. Folic acid comes in tablets (400mcg or 0.4mg per day) and is also found in foods such as green, leafy vegetables, beans, and breads and cereals fortified with folic acid.
- Do not smoke. See your GP (and Chapter 1 of this book) for smoking cessation advice.
- Do not drink more than one or two units of alcohol (see Chapter 1), once or twice a week – or stop altogether.
- Eat a balanced diet, including lots of fruit and vegetables.
- Avoid vitamin A supplements (because high levels of vitamin A can damage the baby's developing nervous system).
- Avoid liver and liver products, such as pâté (because they contain high levels of vitamin A), ripened soft cheese (because it may contain listeria – see below) and raw or undercooked eggs (because of the risk of salmonella, which can cause food poisoning and, rarely, miscarriage).
- Talk to your GP or pharmacist before taking any medicines.

Illness in mother

Q *I am 21 weeks pregnant and suffering from 'flu, and am worried it could affect the health of my unborn baby. Is there any danger?*

A The baby developing in your womb is surprisingly, and wonderfully, resilient and oblivious to things going on in the rest of your body.

There are some viruses that can cross the placenta and cause damage to the unborn baby, such as rubella (German measles). However, these viruses are exceptions, and 'flu is not one of them. It is worth having a check-up with your GP if you have an unexplained fever, and you can ask your GP or midwife to take blood for listeria – a very rare bug that can occasionally cause miscarriage or early labour, but which can be treated with antibiotics if detected.

For colds and 'flu-like illnesses, paracetamol is best for fevers and aches, and is safe to take during pregnancy. Avoid aspirin during pregnancy, especially the later stages as it can affect the baby's heart and circulation.

Not many women manage to survive nine months of pregnancy without succumbing to at least one tummy bug, bad cold or 'flu-like illness – but they are mostly delivered of healthy babies who have obviously not been adversely affected.

Toxoplasmosis

Q *I am 28 weeks pregnant and have two young cats at home. My mother is worried that the cats are a health risk for the baby – is this true? If so, what should I do to minimise the risk?*

A There are two issues when you are pregnant and have cats in the house. The first is whether you are at risk of toxoplasmosis – an infection which can be transmitted to humans from cats' faeces and may damage the unborn child. In fact, most people who have cats for a long time are not particularly at risk, as they often have immunity to the infection already. Everyone who is pregnant should avoid handling cats' litter and be scrupulous about washing their hands after handling raw meat, which is also a source of infection.

The second issue is your baby's safety once it is born. Of course, you will need to ensure that your cats cannot jump on top of the baby and scratch or even suffocate him or her. Pram nets may be handy, but keeping your young baby within view at all times and ensuring the cats cannot get to the baby's crib or carrycot are essential. Many cat lovers have young children, with no harm caused to anyone – it just means being a bit more careful than usual.

Down's syndrome

Q *I am 12 weeks pregnant and recently had an ultrasound scan to check the baby. They told me that the back of the baby's neck is too thick and this can be a sign of Down's syndrome. The blood test I had to check for Down's was normal. I have an appointment with the specialist later this week but am confused about the contradiction. What do you think is a definitive test?*

A Scans and blood tests can provide clues, but they are not definitive. The nuchal fold scan is the measurement of the back of the baby's neck, done on ultrasound scan, that you refer to. It can indicate a suspicion of Down's syndrome or other rarer chromosomal abnormalities, but you will not know for certain until you have a test to sample the baby's cells (CVS or amniocentesis). This is what you will be offered when you see the doctor or midwife at your next appointment, and the chances are it will show that your baby has normal chromosomes. Doctors call abnormal results that turn out to be OK 'false-positives'. For the person on the other end of the test, it is an awful fright over nothing.

Genetic counselling

Q *My husband and I are fit and well and I am happily pregnant with our first child. However, a first cousin of mine had a child who had severe problems from birth and died before the age of five. My mother mentioned this to me and wondered whether I should see a specialist before my own baby is born. I am rather worried now. What do you think I should do?*

A Genetic counselling is a service available in every region of the country, usually based in a large district general hospital or attached to a teaching hospital. You can be referred by your GP if you have concerns about conditions or diseases that appear to run in your family or if you or one of your family are found to be carrying or suffering from a disease that can be inherited.

It is possible that seeing a genetic counsellor would put your mind at rest, but he or she will only be able to give you an assessment of the risk; not a cast-iron guarantee that all will be well. Before you see anyone you need to get more information: for example, the name of any condition or syndrome that the baby had and whether any other family members have experienced similar tragedies.

The counsellor will need to know whether the diagnosis was made without any shadow of a doubt, and as much information as possible about the condition or disease. This information should be contained in hospital letters from specialists, which your GP can send with the referral letter. If you can sketch out a family tree with the ages at which family members died and the cause, if known, it will be extremely helpful.

The counsellor will then put together all this information to give you an idea of the risk to you and other family members of inheriting the disease. Depending on the condition and the implications of the advice you are given, you may want further sessions and psychological support. You may be advised to see a specific specialist, and may want to get in touch with a self-help group, if one exists for that condition. The whole process can be either reassuring, initially devastating, or somewhere in between – depending on what the advice is. Even the worst-case scenario does not always happen and people are often amazed by their own capacity to rally and get on with life, even if they feel they have a sword of Damocles hanging over them.

Morning sickness

Q *I am two months pregnant and I can't cope with the morning sickness. Mine actually lasts most of the day and is making me feel wretched. I don't want to take any drugs if I can avoid it, but I don't think I can cope with this much longer. Is there anything I can do about it?*

A Nausea is very common in the first three months of pregnancy, and is due to the rising hormone levels that are necessary to keep the pregnancy going. You can take comfort from the fact that it usually passes after the first 12 weeks, but for some women it can certainly be very debilitating.

Try eating little and often, avoid the more wacky cravings like pickled eggs, which might make anyone nauseous, and don't get too tired. Ginger helps some people. Acupuncture has been shown to help and is safe in pregnancy.

If vomiting becomes so severe that you are becoming weak, losing weight or are worried, then drug treatment may be advised. This could be antihistamines, which are usually used for allergic reactions, or a drug called promethazine (Avomine), which is used for travel sickness and is considered to be safe in pregnancy.

Nausea can be a sign of a urinary infection, whether you are pregnant or not, so you could take a urine sample to your GP or midwife to be checked.

Pubic pain

Q *I am six months pregnant and in more pain than I could ever have imagined. It feels as though my pubic bone is going to split in half. I get a shooting pain through the pubic bone, round my whole pelvis and in my inner thighs, and a persistent ache in my lower back. It is making me terrified of going into labour – I'm in so much pain already I don't think I could take any more. My GP and midwife have suggested paracetamol and hot baths and don't seem able to come up with anything else. Can you help?*

A Your condition has a name – diastasis symphysis pubis (DSP) – but no known cure. It is common, frightening and painful. The pain can persist for a few weeks after birth but almost always gradually improves after that. Some women are helped by acupuncture; others by physiotherapy. Paracetamol is a painkiller that is safe in pregnancy.

Water birth

Q *I am expecting my first baby in three months and am very keen to have a water birth. My brother-in-law, who works as a gynaecologist in the USA, said that he thinks I'm mad and would be endangering the baby. Is he right – is there any danger?*

A Recent evidence suggests that if you are enjoying a normal pregnancy and are considered at low risk of any complications, water births are as safe as any other method. You will be in a minority – only 2,000 deliveries a year, or just over half a per cent of all deliveries in England and Wales, are water births. Over the two-year study period in 1998, no deaths were directly attributable to the baby having been born in water. This is one to discuss with your midwife or obstetrician, but provided you remain at low risk of complications water birth should be a safe option for you.

Babies and toddlers

Funny-looking genitals

Q *My baby girl is just four days old, and I am worried about the appearance of her vaginal 'lips'. They are very large and look swollen. Should I be concerned?*

A The vaginal lips, or labia, are often swollen in baby girls and can remain so for up to six weeks. Gradually, they will become less swollen-looking and red. The effect is caused by the female hormones that were circulating during your pregnancy, and which have crossed the placenta and affected her genitals. After birth, these hormone levels drop. Some baby girls also get a small amount of vaginal bleeding as a result of the hormone levels having been high and then falling rapidly.

Q *My baby boy is now three months old. He's a very chubby and cheerful soul. The thing that worries me is that his penis seems tiny and almost buried. I'm relieved that we didn't want to have him circumcised – I don't think they would have been able to find it! He seems able to wee all right, but I'm worried about his future as a man. Do you have any advice?*

A Chubby boys often appear to have tiny penises. The reason is just that the pad of fat over their pubic bone (suprapubic fat pad) rather engulfs their member, which is almost certainly no smaller than any other three-month-old's. As he gets leaner, his penis will emerge from the surrounding fat. At puberty, the penis grows and thickens and he will doubtless be able to hold his head up in the changing room.

Cot death

Q *My first baby, a lovely little boy, is now six weeks old. I am absolutely paranoid about cot death. Can you tell me more about it and how I can minimise any risk to my baby?*

A The joy of having a baby is always tempered by the very natural anxieties that can often seem overwhelming, but which lessen with every passing month in which no devastating tragedy has occurred. It is true that cot death claims the lives of eight babies a week in the UK, but that still makes it a rare event. Cot death (or sudden infant death syndrome) is the name given to sudden, unexpected death of a baby. It can occur anywhere, not necessarily in the cot. There are no signs, no warnings and no products available that reliably help to detect its onset. The introduction of a campaign by the Foundation for the Study of Infant Deaths★ in 1991 has halved the number of cot deaths. Although the cause of cot deaths remains unclear, the following measures can help to prevent it:

- place your baby on his or her back to sleep
- stop smoking in pregnancy – fathers too
- do not let anyone smoke in the same room as your baby
- do not let your baby get too hot or cold
- keep your baby's head uncovered – place him or her in the 'feet to foot' position (with the baby's feet touching the foot of the cot) to prevent wriggling down under the covers
- if your baby is unwell, seek medical advice promptly.

MMR vaccination

Q *We have a daughter who has just reached her first birthday. With that date came the inevitable invitation for the MMR jab, a prospect we do not relish. We did hear that in France the vaccines are available in their constituent parts, which we would prefer. Could you tell me whether you know these vaccines to be available individually and, if so, whether they are available in the UK?*

A After the panic generated by claims published in early 2001 by a team at the Royal Free Hospital in London, your concern about MMR (measles, mumps and rubella) is understandable. The study suggested that MMR causes autism and Crohn's disease, a serious bowel disorder. However, the suggested link has not been supported by any other studies or papers (the most prominent of which was published in September 2001 – see 'Autism' in Chapter 2 for details), and there is no evidence to suggest that giving the three components of the MMR jab separately makes them safer, more effective or less likely to cause side-effects – in fact, quite the reverse.

You can get the rubella jab on its own in this country, but most doctors and clinics cannot get the measles or mumps jabs separately – and the mumps jab on its own is less effective than the mumps strain in the MMR. Rumour has it that small quantities of the measles and mumps jabs are being brought into the UK in ice-boxes by doctors returning from France. There are also reports that some private paediatricians are giving the jabs separately because parents have made it clear that it's that or nothing. There is an argument that the jabs should be offered separately to those who want it; but on balance the single MMR is probably the best option.

(See Chapters 1 and 2 for more about vaccination concerns and autism respectively.)

Slow to begin talking

Q *My two-year-old son isn't really talking much, and his 18-month-old cousin says much more than he does. My health visitor agreed that my son should be saying a few words by now, but said that boys often speak later than girls. Is this the case and should I be worried?*

A Two-year-olds can usually join two or three words together, and often babble incessantly. They can generally ask for a drink, snacks or the toilet, and will mimic your speech. Some children speak less, and later, than others, and follow-up studies show that they do just as well in later life as early talkers.

The first step is always to make sure your child can hear properly, and arrange hearing tests with your GP if you are concerned. If your son plays imaginatively, interacts with you and other adults and children, can walk, run and kick a ball and understands what you say to him, he is unlikely to have any developmental delay or autism, but a formal assessment by a community paediatrician may be reassuring. Your child will benefit from every moment you spend reading to him and talking to him, and you may find that attending a playgroup or nursery will help to develop his speech.

It is often said that boys tend to talk later than girls, but there is quite a wide variation between the ages at which different children start to say individual words (generally between 18 months and two-and-a-half years), and a clear difference between the sexes is hard to demonstrate.

School-age children

Head lice

Q *My children have had a lot of trouble with head lice recently and I am determined to get rid of the problem before they go back to school. What is the best way to go about it?*

A There are a number of myths about head lice, which should be put straight. First: there is no evidence that lice prefer clean to dirty hair. Second: they may be itchy and unpleasant, but lice are not dangerous to health. Third: just because you can see nits does not mean there is still active infection – the nits may remain visible for weeks after being killed by treatment.

Using conditioner to make the hair slippery and then combing with a nit comb is advised, though evidence that it works is limited. The various insecticide lotions and shampoos that contain permethrin (e.g. Lyclear) and malathion (e.g. Prioderm) probably work, but the research is flawed and the lice are developing resistance to all the chemicals in common usage. Worries about the safety of malathion, which is an organophosphate (and thought to increase the risk of cancers), have not been confirmed by scientists. Herbal treatments may work but have not been evaluated.

There is no one effective solution, therefore. Conditioner and combing is a good measure but the chemicals are still more reliable to eradicate nits once your child has them.

Molluscum

Q *My children are plagued, as are many others in their school, by warts. Our GP says it's a virus called molluscum contagiosum, and that other than lancing the warts and dabbing them with iodine – which sounds rather brutal – there is nothing you can do. Is there anything you could recommend? Are there any homeopathic remedies that might help?*

A Molluscum have joined head lice, threadworm (see Chapter 7) and verrucas as a seemingly inevitable rite of passage through our nurseries and primary schools. One approach is to leave them alone; like verrucas and other warts, the body eventually fights off the virus that causes them, and they drop off and disappear. However, children who are prone to eczema may get irritating patches of eczema round their molluscum, which can become infected, and spread easily to other family members and children at school.

There is no one anti-molluscum drug that works. Old-fashioned methods of piercing each spot and applying a corrosive chemical like phenol, or freezing them off with liquid nitrogen, are painful, and the phenol method may cause scarring. One method is to apply a cream called EMLA under clingfilm or a similar dressing for an hour to numb the skin and then scoop out the molluscum (curettage). There is also an investigation into whether imiquimod (Aldara) cream, which is used to treat genital and anal warts, works against molluscum. It is used by some specialists, though it is not licensed for use in children. Homeopaths say that taking one thuja tablet a day for a week helps with many molluscum cases and is safe for all ages. Thuja is widely available in pharmacies and health food shops.

Chickenpox

Q *My daughter has chickenpox, and several people are concerned that they could contract shingles from contact with her. What is the connection between chickenpox and shingles?*

A You cannot catch shingles from chickenpox. You can only catch chickenpox from chickenpox, and if you had chickenpox as a child you remain immune forever, in most cases. Moreover, over 85 per cent of adults in the UK are immune to chickenpox, even if they do not remember having had it as a child.

Shingles is not caught from anyone. It is a reactivation of your own chickenpox, which can be stored in cells in your spinal cord for many years. Stress and ill-health may trigger shingles but often there is no rhyme or reason. Nobody need avoid your daughter except pregnant women who have never had chickenpox (as chickenpox in pregnancy may possibly harm an unborn baby), newborn babies and those with impaired immune systems who think they may not be immune to chickenpox.

Persistent colds

Q *My child has had one cold after another since the winter. He is going on an Outward Bound course with his school soon and is likely to get wet through while canoeing, and they sometimes walk around for hours in wet clothes. Is this a serious concern? Should I be careful and insist the school let him change?*

A We get more colds in the winter than the summer because we spend more time huddled together indoors breathing one another's bugs. Also, the cycle of viruses that cause colds changes as the temperature does, so we often get colds as the seasons change.

Severe exposure to cold can impair the immune system and make us prone to severe infections. But even the unpredictable British summer is not usually that bad, so there is no need to worry too much. Your son is probably less likely to catch a bad cold at the Outward Bound course than shut up all day in a stuffy classroom.

Meningitis C vaccination

Q *My daughter is due for her meningitis vaccination next week. I have read reports of serious side-effects, which have me worried. What is the evidence for these effects, and is there any risk of her developing actual meningitis?*

A The meningitis C vaccine is not a live vaccine and definitely cannot cause meningitis or septicaemia (blood poisoning). The vaccine is made by combining the bacterium's sugar coating with a protein, and the injection, which is safe for babies from two months old, gives long-lasting immunity. The jab cannot kill your child but the infection can. Over 60,000 doses have been given worldwide without serious reactions, and it is estimated that 200 children's lives are saved in the UK each year as a result of the vaccination programme.

Your daughter should not have the jab at school if she has a high temperature that day or has had a previous serious reaction to any jab. In those cases, you should discuss the matter first with your GP. Otherwise she will be fine, although the jab does cause redness and swelling of the arm in around 24 per cent of children, and about 10 per cent get a headache. However, these symptoms are preferable by far to the disease itself.

Undescended testicles

Q *At nine years old, my son had two operations to bring down his undescended testicles. Now he is almost 14, but I notice little or no growth in his genitals. A male hormone treatment has been suggested. Is this safe and effective? Is there any alternative treatment?*

A Your son had his operation a little later than is ideal. Although baby boys should be checked routinely at birth, six weeks, seven months and three years old, undescended testicles are sometimes still missed. If the problem is detected in early childhood, most specialists would advise the operation to bring down and fix the testicles in the scrotum at around the age of two, if not before.

The testicles (or testes) develop in the abdominal cavity of baby boys while they are still in the womb, and they are supposed to descend into the scrotum just before birth. The scrotum keeps them cool, which is important for the formation of sperm. Most boys can easily draw up the testes into the groin – if they are cold, for example. This is different from undescended or maldescended (partially descended) testicles, which occur in 2 per cent of boys and means that the testes never descended fully into the scrotum. The right testicle is more commonly affected than the left, and one or both testes may fail to descend properly into the scrotum. Instead, they might lie anywhere along the route that the testes take to reach the scrotum, most commonly in the groin creases.

Undescended testes are more prone to being damaged during accidents, to torsion and to developing testicular cancer (see Chapter 4 for more about these). They are more likely to be abnormal, and that may imply problems in producing sperm later in life.

However, puberty, male characteristics and the ability to have a full sex life should not be jeopardised. Huge advances in male fertility treatment mean that, even if his fertility is impaired, he should still be able to father children. Boys enter puberty at different ages and hormonal treatment is very rarely necessary. Ask your GP for referral to a paediatric endocrinologist for an expert opinion before going ahead with any such treatment.

Smallness

Q *My son is the smallest in his class and it is beginning to get to him. His mother and I are both of average height and were not particularly small as children. He eats well and is very active and fit, but I'm beginning to get anxious on his behalf. Is there anything we can do?*

A Unless your son has an underlying condition limiting his growth, which is rare, he is likely to end up being average height. You need to know whether he is growing at a normal rate ('growth velocity'). Ask your GP to accurately weigh and measure him and plot the results on up-to-date growth charts, which allow a graph of his height and weight to be drawn as he gets older. If your son is especially short (in the smallest 0.4 per cent for his age), or if he appears not to be thriving, your GP will refer you to a growth specialist. If he is small, but repeat measurements in six months' time show that he is growing at normal growth velocity, you can all be reassured. You will be able to explain to your son that he is likely to be at least as tall as his dad, and also that the boys who are tall now may end up as smallish adults – they may go into puberty earlier and stop growing sooner than smaller boys. Listen to his concerns and act promptly if there is any bullying – young boys are very size-sensitive.

Useful information is available from the Child Growth Foundation.★

Bed-wetting (enuresis)

Q *My eight-year-old son still wets the bed. In every other area of his life he is thriving and he never wets himself during the day. I have tried cutting out drinks in the evening and lifting him up from his bed to go to the toilet before we go to sleep, but he is still drenched every morning. He has got a school trip in a few months' time and we really want to solve the problem before he goes. What do you suggest?*

A Bed-wetting is a very common problem, especially for boys. It is also known to be an inherited tendency. For boys who have never been fully dry at night, there is rarely any particular emotional problem – but children who suddenly start wetting the bed are more likely to be worrying about something, and it is a good idea to ask them about what it might be and to talk to their teachers to try to find the cause. For some children, bed-wetting can be part of a more widespread delay in development, and they may wet themselves during the day as well.

For boys like your son who have always wet the bed, it is unlikely that you will identify any particular cause. It would be useful to take him to your GP to have a urine test just to check for any urine infection, which could cause temporary incontinence.

A religiously kept star-chart can work wonders. For example, award a daily coloured star for a dry night, and a gold star for a full week. Agree terms and rewards for a gold star in advance. If that does not work, ask your GP for referral to a clinic that can provide you with a bed-wetting alarm. The alarm lies on the sheet or bedclothes and goes off when in contact with liquid. This wakes your child, who then needs to change the bedclothes, either with you or on his own if possible. (It is the negative effect of having to wake up and change the bed that is supposed to teach him not to wet the bed, rather than any mysterious effect of the bell.) A desmopressin nasal spray or tablets is a very effective short-term way of stopping bed-wetting for school trips, etc. It acts on a hormone released by the brain, which prevents the child from producing urine for a few hours at a time.

Further advice is available from the Enuresis Resource and Information Centre (ERIC).*

Dyspraxia

Q *My nine-year-old son has been diagnosed as dyspraxic, after having social and educational problems at school. What exactly is dyspraxia, how can I get help, and is evening primrose oil, mentioned by a friend, any use?*

A Dyspraxia is an increasingly well-recognised condition that affects children, especially boys. It is a developmental problem thought to be caused by a relative immaturity of the brain which means that some messages are not transmitted properly from the brain to the body. It is said that 2 per cent of the population may be dyspraxic, and over 70 per cent of them are male. Parents may notice that dyspraxic toddlers are slow to feed themselves with a spoon or to learn to dress themselves. As the children grow older they may seen awkward and clumsy. They may walk as if they were about to trip over and find it hard to throw and catch balls, ride bikes, hop or control a pen well enough to write neatly. Their learning may be delayed and their speech may be unclear; moreover, certain behavioural traits including phobias and obsessive rituals may make dyspraxic children hard to cope with. The children may not fit in well at school and may be the subject of bullying, and their behaviour may seem immature compared with that of their peers.

You are fortunate that your son has been diagnosed, because early intervention will improve his outlook. Occupational therapists, physiotherapists and extra help at school can all help him to learn the skills he needs. Evening primrose oil and cod liver oil are sources of a fatty acid (EPA), known to be involved in the development and functioning of our nervous system. Given in the recommended doses, they will not cause any harm, although firm evidence of their benefits in dyspraxia is still awaited.

Advice and support is available from the Dyspraxia Foundation.★

Hyperactivity

Q *I have been called into school countless times about my eight-year-old son, who fidgets and interrupts the teacher, seemingly all the time. The headteacher suggested that I get him assessed to see if he is hyperactive. He is a great kid at home and I have no problems with him at all. What does hyperactivity mean and how would I know if he needs help?*

A Hyperactivity is now called attention deficit hyperactivity disorder (ADHD). It is usually diagnosed in childhood although it may be missed until the individual affected is an adult. It interferes with normal learning, development and behaviour and is similar to dyspraxia (see above) in that it appears to be caused by an immature development of parts of the brain. Up to one in 20 children are said to have the disorder; more boys than girls are affected.

ADHD leads to an inability to concentrate and a tendency to impulsive behaviour that can be hard for others to cope with. Children with ADHD cannot sit still for long. They get up and walk around when other children remain seated as told, fidget endlessly and cannot easily listen to instructions or focus on a particular task. They may find it hard to pick up normal conversational cues so they interrupt inappropriately and may tell jokes that the other kids do not find funny.

This situation causes the child frustration which may be manifest as temper tantrums.

It is important to have a detailed professional assessment and to exclude other possible causes, such as thyroid disorders, autism, illicit drugs (such as glue and other solvents), anxiety and depression. (See Chapters 1 and 2 for more about these.) When a child is much better in one setting (e.g. home), than another (e.g. school), it is particularly necessary to identify the factors that are contributing to the problem. Your son may be being bullied by other children (or even a teacher), or being set inappropriately hard or easy work, or feel anxious about a perceived threat such as SATS exams.

If ADHD is confirmed, treatment includes a programme of behavioural therapy to set goals and reward positive behaviour. Family therapy is sometimes helpful. Medication, chiefly the amphetamine-like drug methylphenidate (Ritalin) can be useful for some children, though its use must be carefully monitored as it can cause weight loss. Some children benefit from cutting out sweets and convenience foods with lots of additives. In that case, help from a dietician is essential as growing children must not be placed on highly restrictive diets.

It is best if you can continue to work closely with the school so that your son feels he is being well supported and that all the adults he knows are pulling in the same direction on his behalf.

Further information is available from the ADHD Information Service.★

Unhappy at school

Q *My 12-year-old daughter has become very withdrawn, difficult to communicate with, and occasionally hostile. She transferred to secondary school recently and doesn't seem to have made new friends. I have asked her whether she is being bullied but she tells me to shut up. Is there anything I can do?*

A It is such a hard transition when children start secondary school. They often have to make new friends, find their way round a school which is almost always far larger than their primary school, cope with a host of new subjects and generally stand on their own two feet with alarming suddenness. In fact, it is a wonder that most cope as well as they do. It is also hard for parents, many of whom were used to chatting at the school gates and being very involved in their child's primary school. Most secondary schools are far less accessible to parents.

Children seem to bring friends home from secondary school less than from primary school; they may be scattered further afield, or have too much homework, or there may just be a teenage culture, which develops higher up the school, of going out rather than staying in with friends.

Your daughter is becoming a teenager and asserting her own individuality and independence. She may not want to be quizzed in too much detail. A shared outing doing something she enjoys is a better forum for open discussion than, for example, an intense encounter in the kitchen. Look for signs of distress: weight loss, drug use (see Chapter 1), negativity and lack of enjoyment in anything, or sleep disturbance (see Chapter 2 for more about depression and anxiety).

Book an appointment to see your daughter's teacher and find out whether there is a system within the school offering pastoral care to keep an informal eye on her. You may be picking up genuine unease in your daughter but you may also be projecting some of your own anxiety about her transition into a more adult world which is outside of your control. Her teacher may be able to ask her some open questions to elicit whether she is having a bad experience at school or not. The school ought to have an anti-bullying policy and you may want to find out more about it so that you can support its implementation on behalf of your daughter, if necessary.

You can leave the door open for your daughter by reassuring her of your love, and letting her know that she can tell you anything, any time. You cannot solve all teenage angst, but unconditional love, some clear and fair boundaries and an open channel of communication prevents a lot of parent–teenager conflict.

Addresses and web sites

Addresses

Action on Smoking and Health (ASH)
102 Clifton Street
London EC2A 4HW
Tel: 020-7739 5902
Fax: 020-7613 0531
Email: action.smoking.health@
dial.pipex.com
Web site: www.ash.org.uk

Adoption Information Line
193 Market Street
Hyde
Cheshire SK14 1HF
Tel: (0800) 783 4086 (9am–9pm)
Email: office@adoption.org.uk,
office@fostering.org.uk
Web sites: www.adoption.org.uk,
www.fostering.org.uk

Alcoholics Anonymous (AA)
General Service Office
P.O. Box 1
Stonebow House
Stonebow
York YO1 7NJ
Tel: (01904) 644026
Fax: (01904) 629091
Web site: www.alcoholics-
anonymous.org.uk
*Local groups are listed in the telephone
directory under 'Alcoholics Anonymous'*

Al-Anon Family Groups UK
61 Great Dover Street
London SE1 4YF
Tel: 020-7403 0888 (10am–10pm)
Fax: 020-7378 9910
*The above number is a confidential
helpline for families and friends of addicts;
callers can be directed to their local group*

Aromatherapy Organisations Council
P.O. Box 19834
London SE25 6WF
*Send an A4 SAE for a general
information boolet*

Association for Postnatal Illness (APNI)
145 Dawes Road
Fulham
London SW6 7EB
Tel: 020-7386 0868
Fax: 020-7386 8885
Email: info@apni.org
Web site: www.apni.org

Association of Reflexologists
27 Old Gloucester Street
London WC1N 3XX
Tel: (08705) 673320
Fax: (01989) 567676
Email: aor@reflexology.org
Web site: www.aor.org.uk

**Attention Deficit Hyperactivity
Disorder (ADHD) Information
Service**
P.O. Box 340
Edgware
Middlesex HA8 9HL
Tel: 020-8905 2013
Fax: 020-8386 6466
Email: addiss@compuserve.com
Web site: www.adhd.co.uk

Barnardo's
Tanners Lane
Barkingside, Ilford
Essex IG6 1QG
Tel: 020-8550 8822
Fax: 020-8551 6870
Email: dorothy.howes@
barnardos.org.uk
Web site: www.barnardos.org.uk
*Helps children with problems such as
disability, educational difficulties, sexual,
physical or emotional abuse, poverty or
life-threatening illness such as
HIV/AIDS*

The Beaumont Trust
BM Charity
London WC1N 3XX
Helpline: (07000) 287878
(Tues & Thurs 7–11 pm)
Email: bmonttrust@aol.com
Web site: hometown.aol.com/
bmonttrust/Index1.htm
*Assists transvestites, transsexuals, and
their friends and families through advice,
support groups and literature*

British Acupuncture Council (BAC)
63 Jeddo Road
London W12 9HQ
Tel: 020-8735 0400
Fax: 020-8735 0404
Email: info@acupuncture.org.uk
Web site: www.acupuncture.org.uk

**British Association of Aesthetic
Plastic Surgeons (BAAPS)**
Royal College of Surgeons
35–43 Lincoln's Inn Fields
London WC2A 3PN
Tel: 020-7405 2234
Fax: 020-7430 1840
Email: info@baaps.org.uk
Web site: www.baaps.org.uk

**British Association of Plastic
Surgeons (BAPS)**
Royal College of Surgeons
35–43 Lincoln's Inn Fields
London WC2A 3PN
Tel: 020-7831 5161
Fax: 020-7831 4041
Email: secretariat@baps.co.uk
Web site: www.baps.co.uk

**British Association of Sexual and
Marital Therapy**
P.O. Box 62
Sheffield S10 3TS
*A list of sexual and relationships clinics is
available from this address*

British Heart Foundation
14 Fitzhardinge Street
London W1H 6DH
Tel: 020-7487 7125
Web site: www.bhf.org.uk
*Details of your local cardiac care group
available from the above number*

British Homoeopathic Association
15 Clerkenwell Close
London EC1R 0AA
Tel: 020-7566 7800
Fax: 020-7566 7815
Email: info@homoeopathy.org.uk
Web site: www.homoeopathy.org.uk

British Massage Therapy Council
17 Rymers Lane
Oxford OX4 3JU
Tel: (01865) 774123
Email: enquiries@bmtc.co.uk
Web site: www.bmtc.co.uk

British Pregnancy Advisory Service (BPAS)
Austy Manor
Wootton Wawen
Solihull
West Midlands B95 6BX
Tel: (01564) 793225
Actionline (for abortion):
(08457) 304030
Fax: (01564) 794935
Email: comm@bpas.org
Web site: www.bpas.org

British Stammering Association
15 Old Ford Road
London E2 9PJ
Tel: 020-8983 1003
Helpline: (0845) 603 2001
Fax: 020-8983 3591
Email: mail@stammering.org
Web site: www.stammering.org

British Tinnitus Association
4th Floor
White Building
Fitzalan Square
Sheffield S1 2AZ
Tel: 0114-279 6600
Helpline: (08000) 180527
Fax: 0114-279 6222
Email: enquiries@tinnitus.org.uk
Web site: www.tinnitus.org.uk

Brook Advisory Centres
421 Highgate Studios
53–79 Highgate Road
London NW5 1TL
Tel: (0800) 018 5023
Advice on sexual matters for the under-25s. Telephone numbers of local centres are available from the above number

CancerBACUP
3 Bath Place
Rivington Street
London EC2A 3JR
Information: 020-7613 2121
Tel: (0808) 800 1234 (Mon–Fri 9am–7pm)
Fax: 020-7696 9002
Email: info@cancerbacup.org
Web site: www.cancerbacup.org

Cancer Research Campaign
10 Cambridge Terrace
London NW1 4JL
Tel: 020-7224 1333
Fax: 020-7487 4310
Web site: www.crc.org.uk

CHILD (National Infertility Support Network)
Charter House
43 St Leonards Road
Bexhill-on-Sea
East Sussex TN40 1JA
Tel: (01424) 732361
Fax: (01424) 731858
Email: office@child.org.uk
Web site: www.child.org.uk

Child Growth Foundation
2 Mayfield Avenue
Chiswick
London W4 1PW
Tel: 020-8994 7625/8995 0257
Fax: 020-8995 9075
Email: cgflondon@aol.com
Web site: www.cgf.org.uk

Childline
Studd Street
London N1 0QW
Tel: 020-7239 1000
Childline: (0800) 1111
Fax: 020-7239 1001
Email: info@childline.org.uk
Web site: www.childline.org.uk

Continence Foundation
307 Hatton Square
16 Baldwins Gardens
London EC1N 7RJ
Incontinence helpline:
020-7831 9831 (Mon–Fri
9.30am–4.30pm)
Email: continence-help@
dial.pipex.com
Web site:
www.continencefoundation.org.uk

Depression Alliance
35 Westminster Bridge Road
London SE1 7JB
Tel: 020-7633 0557
Helpline: 020-7633 0101
(Mon–Fri 6–9pm)
Fax: 020-7633 0559
Web site:
www.depressionalliance.org

The Dyscovery Centre
4a Church Road
Whitchurch
Cardiff CF14 2DZ
Tel: 029-2062 8222
Fax: 029-2062 8333
Email: dyscoverycentre@btclick.com
Web site: www.dyscovery.co.uk
*Addresses the needs of children and adults
with a wide range of living and learning
difficulties, providing assessment,
treatment, support and practical advice*

Dyspraxia Foundation
8 West Alley
Hitchin
Hertfordshire SG5 1EG
Helpline: (01462) 454986
Fax: (01462) 455052
Email:
admin@dyspraxiafoundation.org.uk
Web site:
www.dyspraxiafoundation.org.uk

Eating Disorders Association
1st Floor
Wensum House
103 Prince of Wales Road
Norwich NR1 1DW
Adult advice line:
(01603) 621414 (9am–6.30pm)
Youth line: (01603) 765050 (4–6pm)
Fax: (01603) 664915
Email: info@edauk.com
Web site: www.edauk.com

**Enuresis Resource and Information
Centre (ERIC)**
34 Old School House
Britannia Road
Kingswood
Bristol BS15 8DB
Tel: 0117-960 3060
Fax: 0117-960 0401
Email: info@eric.org.uk
Web site: www.eric.org.uk

Family Matters
13 Wrotham Road
Gravesend
Kent DA11 0PA
Tel: (01474) 536661
Fax: (01474) 536669
Helpline: (0808) 808 8080 (variable
hours)
Email: admin.grfm@btclick.com
*Aims to relieve the physical and mental
distress of victims of sexual abuse and to
raise awareness of abuse. Can direct
callers to local support groups*

Fertility UK
Clitherow House
1 Blythe Mews
Blythe Road
London W14 0NW
Tel: 020-7371 1341
Fax: 020-7371 4921
Web site: www.fertilityuk.org

Foundation for the Study of Infant Deaths
Artillery House
11–19 Artillery Row
London SW1P 1RT
Tel: 020-7222 8001
24hr helpline: 020-7233 2090
Fax: 020-7222 8002
Email: fsid@sids.org.uk
Web site: www.sids.org.uk

The Fresh Breath Centre
Conan Doyle House
2 Devonshire Place
London W1G 6HJ
Tel: 020-7935 1666
Fax: 020-7935 8225
Email: fresh.breath@virgin.net
Web site: www.freshbreath.co.uk

General Chiropractic Council
3rd Floor, North Wing
344–354 Gray's Inn Road
London WC1X 8BP
Tel: 020-7713 5155
Fax: 020-7713 5844
Email: enquiries@gcc-uk.org
Web site: www.gcc-uk.org

General Council and Register of Naturopaths (GCRN)
Goswell House
2 Goswell Road
Street
BA16 0JG
Tel: (01458) 840072
Fax: (01458) 840075
Email: admin@naturopathy.org.uk
Web site: www.naturopathy.org.uk

Hearing Aid Council
Witan Court
305 Upper Fourth Street
Milton Keynes MK9 1EH
Tel: (01908) 235700
Fax: (01908) 233770
Email:
hac@thehearingaidcouncil.org.uk
Web site:
www.thehearingaidcouncil.org.uk

Hearing Concern
7–11 Armstrong Road
London W3 7JL
Tel: 020-8743 1110
Helpline (text and voice):
(08450) 744600
Minicom: 020-8743 9151
Textphone: 020-8742 9151
Email: info@hearingconcern.org.uk
Web site:
www.hearingconcern.org.uk

Herpes Viruses Association
41 North Road
London N7 9DP
Helpline: 020-7609 9061
Web site: www.herpes.org.uk

Human Fertilisation and Embryology Authority (HFEA)
Paxton House
30 Artillery Lane
London E1 7LS
Tel: 020-7377 5077
Fax: 020-7377 1871
Email: admin@hfea.gov.uk
Web site: www.hfea.gov.uk

Incontact
United House
North Road
London N7 9DP
Tel: 020-7700 7035
Email: edu@incontact.org
Web site: www.incontact.
demon.co.uk
A membership organisation run by and
for people with bowel and bladder
problems and their carers

Institute of Psychosexual Medicine
12 Chandos Street
Cavendish Square
London W1G 9DR
Tel: 020-7580 0631
Web site: www.ipm.org.uk

Irritable Bowel Syndrome (IBS)
Network
Northern General Hospital
Herries Road
Sheffield S5 7AU
Tel: 0114-261 1531
Helpline: (01543) 492192
(Mon–Fri 6–8pm, Sat 10am–12pm)
Information and support for IBS sufferers,
their families and carers

Kinesiology Federation
P.O. Box 17153
Edinburgh EH11 3WQ
Tel/Fax: (08700) 113545
Email:
kfadmin@kinesiologyfederation.org
Web site:
www.kinesiologyfederation.org

The London Breath Centre
93 Haverstock Hill
London NW3 4RL
Tel: 020-7586 7237
Fax: 020-7483 1246
Web site: www.fresherbreath.com

Lupus UK
St James's House
Eastern Road
Romford
Essex RM1 3NH
Tel: (01708) 731251

Manic Depression Fellowship
Castle Works
21 St. George's Road
London SE1 6ES
Tel: 020-7793 2600
Fax: 020-7793 2639
Email: mdf@mdf.org.uk
Web site: www.mdf.org.uk

ME Association
4 Corringham Road
Stanford-le-Hope
Essex SS17 0AH
Tel: (01375) 642466
Fax: (01375) 360256
Email: enquiries@
meassociation.org.uk
Web site: www.meassociation.org.uk

Meet A Mum Association (MAMA)
77 Westbury View
Peasedown St John
Bath BA2 8TZ
Tel: (01761) 433598
Helpline: 020-8768 0123
(Mon–Fri 7–10pm)
Email: meet-a-mum-
assoc@ blueyonder.co.uk
Web site: www.mama.org.uk
Self-help groups for mothers with small
children

Migraine Action Association
178a High Road
Byfleet, West Byfleet
Surrey KT14 7ED
Tel: (01932) 352468
Fax: (01932) 351257
Email: info@migraine.org.uk
Web site: www.migraine.org.uk

MIND
Granta House
15–19 Broadway
Stratford
London E15 4BQ
Tel: 020-8519 2122
Fax: 020-8522 1725
Email: contact@mind.org.uk
Web site: www.mind.org.uk
*Local groups offer a range of support
services including a legal service*

MoreToLife
114 Lichfield Street
Walsall WS1 1SZ
Tel: (0705) 003 7905 (local rate)
Fax: (01922) 640070
Email: info@moretolife.co.uk
Web site: www.moretolife.co.uk

National AIDS helpline
Tel: (0800) 567123 (24 hours)
Minicom: (0800) 521361
(10am–10pm)

**National Association for
Premenstrual Syndrome (NAPS)**
7 Swifts Court
High Street
Seal
Kent TN15 0EG
Tel/Fax: (01732) 760011
Helpline (01732) 760012
Email: contact@pms.org.uk
Web site: www.pms.org.uk

National Autistic Society
393 City Road
London EC1V 1NG
Tel: 020-7833 2299
Helpline: (0870) 600 8585
(Mon–Fri 10am–4pm)
Fax: 020-7833 9666
Email: nas@nas.org.uk
Web site: www.nas.org.uk
*Deals with all aspects of autism and
Asperger's syndrome*

National Drugs Helpline
(0800) 776600
*This number is free, confidential and will
not appear on your phone bill*

National Eczema Society
Hill House
Highgate Hill
London N19 5NA
Tel: 020-7281 3553
Fax: 020-7281 6395
Helpline: (0870) 241 3604
(Mon–Fri 1–4pm)
Web site: www.eczema.org

**National Federation of Spiritual
Healers**
Old Manor Farm Studio
Church Street
Sunbury-on-Thames
Middlesex TW16 6RG
Tel: (01932) 783164
Fax: (01932) 779648
Email: office@nfsh.org.uk
Web site: www.nfsh.org.uk

**National Institute of Medical
Herbalists (NIMH)**
56 Long Brook Street
Exeter
Devon EX4 6AH
Tel: (01392) 426022
Fax: (01392) 498963
Email: nimh@ukexeter.
freeserve.co.uk
Web site: www.NIMH.org.uk

**National Osteoporosis Society
(NOS)**
P.O. Box 10
Radstock
Bath BA3 3YB
Tel (general enquiries):
(01761) 471771
Helpline (medical queries):
(01761) 472721
Fax: (01761) 471104
Email: info@nos.org.uk
Web site: www.nos.org.uk

National Phobic Society
Zion Community Resource Centre
339 Stretford Road
Hulme
Manchester M15 4ZY
Tel: (0870) 770 0456
Fax: 0161-227 9862
Email: natphob.soc@good.co.uk
Web site: www.phobics-society.org.uk

National Register of Hypnotherapists and Psychotherapists (NRHP)
Suite B
12 Cross Street
Nelson
Lancashire BB9 7EN
Tel: (01282) 716839
Fax: (01282) 698633
Email: nrhp@btconnect.com
Web site: www.nrhp.co.uk

National Schizophrenia Fellowship (NSF)
28 Castle Street
Kingston-upon-Thames
Surrey KT1 1SS
Tel: 020-8547 3937
Advice Service: 020-8974 6814
(Mon–Fri 10am–3pm)
Fax: 020-8547 3862
Helps people with a severe mental illness, and their families and carers, through support groups, publications and services in England, Wales and Northern Ireland
The Voices Forum *is part of the NSF and has a number of local groups offering support, friendship and understanding*

National Schizophrenia Fellowship (Scotland)
Claremont House
130 East Claremont Street
Edinburgh EH7 4LB
Tel: 0131-557 8969
Fax: 0131-557 8698
Carelinkline (for Grampian region): (01224) 213034

NHS Direct
Tel: (0845) 4647 (24 hours)
Part of the National Health Service, this is a nurse-led telephone service, providing 24-hour access to information and advice about health, illness and health services

Parents Against Drug Abuse
14 Church Parade
Ellesmere Port
South Wirral CH65 2ER
Tel: 0151-356 1996
Helpline: (08457) 023867
Email: padahelp@btinternet.com
Web site:
www.btinternet.com/~padahelp/

Psoriasis Association
Milton House
7 Milton Street
Northampton NN2 7JG
Tel: (01604) 711129
Fax: (01604) 792894
Email: mail@psoriasis.demon.co.uk

Rape Crisis Federation
7 Mansfield Road
Nottingham NG1 3FB
Tel: 0115-934 8474
Fax: 0115-934 8470
Email: info@rapecrisis.co.uk
Web site: www.rapecrisis.co.uk
Contact for details of your local rape crisis centre

Relate
Herbert Gray College
Little Church Street
Rugby
Warwickshire CV21 3AP
Tel: (01788) 573241
Fax: (01788) 535007
Email: enquiries@national.
relate.org.uk
Web site: www.relate.org.uk
Telephone numbers of local branches are listed in the telephone directory under 'Relate'

Relate (Northern Ireland)
74–76 Dublin Road
Belfast BT2 7HP
Tel: 028-9032 3454
Fax: 028-9031 5298
Email: office@relateni.org
Web site: www.relateni.org/
infopage.htm

Release
388 Old Street
London EC1V 9LT
Tel: 020-7729 9904
(Overnight): 020-7603 8654
Fax: 020-7729 2599
Email: info@release.org.uk
Web site: www.release.org.uk
*Gives advice to drug users, their families
and friends, and specialises in legal issues*

**Royal National Institute for Deaf
People (RNID)**
19–23 Featherstone Street
London EC1Y 8SL
Tel: (0808) 808 0123
Textphone: (0808) 808 9000
Fax: 020-7296 8199
Tinnitus helpline:
(08457) 090210
E-mail: informationline@
rnid.org.uk
Web site: www.rnid.org.uk

The Samaritans
P.O. Box 9090
Stirling FK8 2SA
Helpline: (08457) 909090
Email: jo@samaritans.org
Web site: www.samaritans.org
*Offers support to those who feel suicidal or
despairing; local branch numbers are listed
in the telephone directory*

SANE
First Floor
Cityside House
40 Adler Street
London E1 1EE
Tel: 020-7375 1002
Fax: 020-7375 2162
Saneline: (08457) 678 000
*Offers emotional support and practical
information to sufferers, carers and family
members coping with mental illness*

**The Society of Teachers of the
Alexander Technique**
129 Camden Mews
London NW1 9AH
Tel: 020-7284 3338
Fax: 020-7482 5435
Email: info@stat.org.uk
Web site: www.stat.org.uk

Terence Higgins Trust (THT)
52–54 Gray's Inn Road
London WC1X 8JE
Tel: 020-7831 0330
THT Direct: (0845) 122 1200
Fax: 020-7242 0121
Email: info@tht.org.uk
Web site: www.tht.org.uk
*The leading HIV and AIDS charity in
the UK*

Tourette's Syndrome Association
1st Floor Offices
Old Bank Chambers
London Road
Crowborough
East Sussex TN6 2TT
Helpline: (01892) 669151
Fax: (01892) 663649
Email: enquiries@tsa.org.uk
Web site: www.tsa.org.uk

Triumph Over Phobia (TOP UK)
P.O. Box 1831
Bath BA2 4YW
Tel: (01225) 330353
Fax: (01225) 469212
Email: triumphoverphobia@
compuserve. com
Web site:
www.triumphoverphobia.com

Women's Health
52 Featherstone Street
London EC1Y 8RT
Tel: 020-7251 6333
Helpline: (0845) 125 5254
(Mon–Fri 9.30am–1.30pm)
Minicom: 020-7490 5489
Fax: 020-7250 4152
Email: womenshealth@
pop3.poptel.org.uk
Web site:
www.womenshealthlondon.org.uk
*Health information on gynaecological
health issues*

**Women's Nationwide Cancer
Control Campaign**
WNCCC Cancer Aware
1st Floor, Charity House
14–15 Perseverance Works
London E2 8DD
Tel: 020-7729 4688
Fax: 020-7613 0771
Email: admin@wnccc.org.uk
Web site: www.wnccc.org.uk
*Promotes the prevention and early
detection of cancers affecting women,
offers self-help advice and support groups*

Web sites

Bad Breath Research
www.tau.ac.il/~melros/welcome.html.

Blushing Buyer
www.blushingbuyer.co.uk
Online store for personal health products

British Society of Hearing Aid Audiologists (BHSAA)
www.bshaa.co.uk

Embarrassing Problems
www.embarrassingproblems.co.uk
Advice about embarrassing health problems

CancerHelp UK
www.cancerhelp.org.uk
From the Cancer Research Campaign, a free information service about cancer and cancer care for the general public. Includes sections on causes, warning signs, treatment and reducing the risk of cancer

Channel 4 ('A beginner's guide to coming out')
www.channel4.com/plus/out

The Health Education Board for Scotland (drug misuse information)
www.hebs.scot.nhs.uk/services/drugs

Restless Legs Syndrome Foundation
www.rls.org
A US organisation, with support group contacts in the UK

The Society of Chiropodists and Podiatrists
www.feetforlife.org/

Sun Know How
www.doh.gov.uk/sunknowhow/index.htm
Practical advice from the Department of Health to reduce risk of skin cancer

UK Patient Self-help and Support Groups
www.patient.co.uk/selfhelp

Your Guide to the NHS
www.nhs.uk/nhsguide
Sets out what you can expect from the NHS at present and in the future as improvements to health services are made

Index

antispasmodic drugs 199, 203
anus *see* back passage
Anusol 201
Anusol-HC 201
anxiety 45, 48, 52–3, 57, 72, 218
appendicitis 196
appendix 196
appetite disturbance 46
appetite loss 151
aqueous creams 223, 225, 228
aromatherapy 41
Arret 199, 203, 207
arteries, damaged 11, 12, 34
artificial insemination by husband
    (AIH) 180, 181
Asperger's disorder 43, 55, 65–6
aspirin 32, 70, 140, 252, 271
assertiveness training 55–6
assisted conception 179–81
    artificial insemination by husband
        (AIH) 180, 181
    donor insemination (DI) 180–1,
        182
    egg donation 179, 181
    gamete intrafallopian transfer
        (GIFT) 180, 181
    in-vitro fertilisation (IVF) 179–80,
        181, 182
    intracytoplasmic sperm injection
        (ICSI) 180, 181
    intrauterine/insemination (IUI)
        181
    pronuclear stage embryo transfer
        (PROST) 180, 181
asthma 32
athlete's foot 215
atrophic vaginitis 77, 79
attention deficit hyperactivity
    disorder (ADHD) 284–5
autism 43, 65–8, 277
auto-immune diseases 15, 30
Avloclor 30
Avomine 274
azathioprine 30

babies and toddlers 275–8
    cot death 269, 276
    genitals 275
    slow in talking 277–8
    vaccination 276–7
    see also children
back pain 53
back passage 191
    cracks around 198
    digital rectal examination 124,
        125, 191
    itchy bottom 132, 134, 200–2
    piles 152, 185, 201–2, 204, 205
    rectal bleeding 152, 198, 201,
        202–3, 204–5
    slime or mucus from 197, 204
    warts around 203–4
backache 197
bacterial vaginosis (BV) 94, 100–1,
    131, 132–3, 212, 213
balanitis 100, 110, 114
balanitis xerotica obliterans 115
baldness 243–4
barium enema 191, 206
Bartholin's cyst 136
basal cell carcinomas 236–7
Beau's lines 246
Beconase 266
bed-wetting 282–3
behavioural therapy 44–5
belly-button, protruding 196
benign essential tremor 72
benign positional vertigo (BPV) 254
benign prostatic hypertrophy (BPH)
    123–4
benzoyl peroxide 225, 231
bestiality 106
beta-blockers 52, 53, 54, 56, 90
Betaferon 30
betahistine 262
Betnovate 229
binge eating 58, 59
biofeedback 262
bipolar disease *see* manic depression
birthmarks 232, 238
bisphosphonates 189

streptococcus 69

stress 43, 51, 193–4, 198, 227, 263, 280

see also anxiety; depression

stretch marks 240–1

stroke 11, 17, 32, 34, 170, 171, 207, 253

multi-infarct dementia (MID) 70

risk factors 171

styes 257

sudden infant death syndrome *see* cot death

suicidal thoughts 48, 63

sulfasalazine 199

sumatriptan 253

sunspots 234

support bandages and stockings 229, 240

suppositories 191, 201

Suprefact 141

swallowing, difficulty in 190–3, 194

sweating 13, 52, 55, 72, 208, 209

body odour 217–19

hyperhidrosis 209, 218

night sweats 183, 188

smelly feet 214–17

sympathectomy 209, 216, 219

syndromes

Asperger's disorder 43, 55, 65–6

autism 43, 65–8

obsessive-compulsive disorder (OCD) 45, 48, 64–5

Tietze's syndrome 157

Tourette's syndrome 43, 68–9

toxic shock syndrome 153, 214

syphilis 94, 95, 97–8, 99

Tagamet 90, 127, 194

talking therapies 44–5, 46–7, 57

see also behavioural therapy; cognitive behavioural therapy (CBT); family and marital therapy; psychodynamic psychotherapy

tamoxifen 127

tampon, forgotten 153, 212, 214

tattoos 232–3

tazarotene 228

Tegretol 74, 255

temporal arteritis 256

tension headaches 251

tension-free vaginal tape (TVT) 154

terazosin 124

testicles 114, 117–22

artificial testicles 120

lumps or pain in 117–18, 119, 121

self-examination 122

surgical removal 119, 120

testicular torsion 118

undescended testicles 121, 281–2

testicular cancer 107, 117, 118–22, 281

warning signs 121

testosterone 86, 90, 91, 114, 120, 124, 128, 230

tetanus 36

thread veins 220, 238–9

threadworm 200–1

throat

hoarse 38

mucus, excess 193–4

swallowing 190–3, 194

thrombophlebitis 240

thrombosis 147, 166, 170, 171, 186

deep vein thrombosis 170

thrush 232

in men 100, 108–10

oral thrush 266–7

vaginal thrush 79, 81, 82, 94, 100, 131–2

thuja 279

thyroid 13

overactive 13, 72, 144, 184, 218

underactive 12, 13, 29, 78, 229, 254

thyroid-stimulating hormone (TSH) 13

thyroxine 13

tics 69

Tietze's syndrome 157

tinnitus 262

tiredness/lethargy 13, 15, 28–31, 197